TABLE OF CONTENTS

Vital Sensation Manual

UNIT FOUR:
MIASMS

**Based on
The Sensation Method
& Classical Homeopathy**

Written
by
Melissa Burch, CCH & Susana Aikin, CCH

Edited by Ingrid Dankmeyer, Didi Pershouse and Sharon Willis

Cover Design by Chetana Deorah

Text Design by Janet Innes and George Papargyris

Published by
Inner Health, Inc.
175 Harvey St., #13
Cambridge, MA 02140
(617) 491-3374
melissa@innerhealth.us
www.innerhealth.us

A. NEW INSIGHT INTO MIASMS

Collective susceptibility leading to widespread epidemics are also turbulent surfacing movements of miasm. In this sense, miasms exist in the holographic universal consciousness and therefore affect any and all parts of that universal totality.

Susana Aikin, CCH

Of all complex thinking in homeopathic philosophy, the most challenging concept handed down by Hahnemann to his disciples and students was probably the theory of miasms. Since then and throughout the following centuries, homeopaths have struggled with understanding the theory of miasms and have found the theory difficult to integrate in their daily practice. In the light of such difficulty, many have just followed Hering's attitude of bypassing miasms. He wrote, "What influence can it have whether a physician adopts or rejects the Psoric theory so long as he searches for the most similar medicine possible?" Homeopaths following this approach simply worked to search for the best similimum in each case, ignoring miasms at large. But even when ignored, the theory of miasms doesn't leave the homeopathic community's collective consciousness, and keeps resurfacing intermittently. Surely it is practically impossible to disregard what Hahnemann himself wrote of the theory of miasms: "Of this invaluable discovery, of which the worth to mankind exceeds all else that has ever been discovered by me, and without which all existent Homeopathy remains defective or imperfect ..."

In "Chronic Diseases" published in 1828, Hahnemann proposed the theory that underlying all chronic disease and all susceptibility to sickness exists at a deeper, greater, more ancient layer of disharmony that dictates and directs all other patterns and symptoms of disease in a human being, eventually driving him to physical death. Miasms are underlying rivers of disease that run deep within the human race. It is the genetic or hereditary tendencies in an organism that has a specific type of decay and destruction or disease and suffering. They are the genetic or hereditary tendencies in an organism that lead to specific types of decay, destruction, disease and suffering.

Hahnemann traced three main miasms in humanity after a decade of intense study of patterns of anamnesis in different forms of chronic disease: Psora, Sycosis and Syphilis. Psora he believed to be the most ancient, the "most monstrous chronic miasm." He related it to the 'ancient itch' or scabies and its suppression, and traced its origin back through the history of all nations. Sycosis and Syphilis he related to venereal diseases, gonorrhea and syphilis respectively, and considered them minor in comparison to Psora, which he believed to be the 'only real fundamental cause and producer of all the other forms of disease' (Organon, Aphorism # 80).

Hahnemann thought that miasms arose originally from these strong infectious agents that were suppressed through faulty medical treatment and driven inwards into the organism. This suppression caused a systemic state, which permeated every cell in the body to such an extent that the disease imprint could then be genetically transferred from one generation to the next through heredity.

The subject of miasms became a moral issue among homeopaths because Hahnemann related each miasm to a particular disease (itch, gonorrhea and syphilis), which were associated with 'taints' and 'sins' or faulty behavior in mankind. Kent added to the difficulty through his more fundamental attitudes concerning the theory of miasms and wrote: "…man by his thinking evils and willing falses has entered upon a state wherein he has lost his freedom, his internal order…" This approach narrowed down the deeper understanding of the miasmatic phenomena, which is mostly unrelated to any specific pathology or ideology.

Miasms are, in the most abstract Hahnemannian sense, tendencies in which matter (the physical body) degrades and is eventually destroyed within the parameters of time and space. Therefore, miasms are dynamic energy forces that inform the organism of the pace, mode and depth of its own destructive process. As deep ancient forces, miasms are not only contagious, but also hereditary and 'coexistent with the life force' from birth, or more accurately from conception. They inform the entire system of being: the physical body, the mind, the emotions, the sensations, the spirit. They lay down the patterns of susceptibility of a particular individual, and the paths down which an individual will attract and contract certain maladies and will mandate the pace and modalities in which they will progress. It will also create tendencies that predispose emotions and personality traits; as well as certain delusions and behaviors.

The overall influence of miasms is truly monstrous over human life and unfortunately mostly invisible. They are only partially discernible through acute manifestations of disease and chronic traits of suffering. For this reason Hahnemann termed Psora 'a multi-headed hydra', because it is so difficult to identify it at once in its totality, since its manifestations can be so impossibly diverse and multiple.

Disease, the specific pathology or collections of symptoms is only a smaller partial manifestation of the larger deeper all encompassing miasm that is bound to the life force and permeates all layers of the being. H.C. Allen wrote that disease: "is but the influence of some subversive force, acting in conjunction with the life force, subverting the action and changing the physiological momentum. Thus we can safely say that disease is but a modified mode of motion, a vibratory change." This subversive force is the miasm so that the nature and character of the disease depends on the form of the miasm and its influence on the life force of the individual. From this viewpoint, the study of disease becomes a study into the nature of the miasm present in the organism and the degree of its activity.

Miasms are also not only circumscribed to individual human beings but also affect social groups, such as families or entire societies. We frequently find families manifesting one specific miasm in different ways, or find children in a family expressing the predominant miasm of either the father or the mother. Miasms can also manifest in larger groups such as entire societies. Collective susceptibility leading to widespread epidemics are also turbulent surfacing movements of miasm. In this sense, miasms exist in the holographic universal consciousness and can affect any and all parts of that universal totality.

One of the practical problems inherent in Hahnemann's legacy of miasms is that he left no comprehensive description of any of the miasms or any type of map that would allow his followers to easily explore his enormous discovery. He listed numerous symptoms of Psora and elaborated long lists of remedies belonging mostly to the Psoric miasm, and shorter lists for Sycotic and Syphilitic miasms.

This situation left the following generations of homeopaths in an awkward position. Some like Boenninghausen tried to follow the Master's work and added more remedies to the lists of miasmatic substances and additional symptoms to the abstract description of miasms. Others like Herring just ignored the miasms altogether. Kent concluded that the theory of miasms did not totally belong to the medical sphere, because "it goes to the very primitive wrong of the human race, the very first sickness of the human race, that is, the spiritual sickness."

Kent influenced the theory of miasms by imbuing it with a religious significance. He described Psora as a state in the human being without which, 'there would be no ground in his economy upon which (disease) would thrive and develop.' This approach created a moralistic view of Psora as a spiritual disease initially brought to man by "the primitive wrong of the human being," nothing less than the original sin. Psora pointed to a separation from nature, a rupture of harmony with the divine, a fall from paradise. The first instance of susceptibility in mankind happened precisely at the very moment of becoming human. Kent's stand further discouraged many homeopaths, mostly sober empirical scientists, from pursuing miasms.

It wasn't until 1944, when the Mexican homeopath, Proceso Ortega published his "Notes on the Miasms" that the whole topic was revitalized. Ortega ascribed very specific characteristics to each miasm. He said the main idea of Psora was inhibition, for Sycosis it was excess and for Syphilis, destruction. Ortega further elaborated on the different miasms as "one state of existence out of the many which can be adopted or produced by this invisible entity…" He once more insisted that treating miasms should be the ultimate concern of the physician, because it brings a deep understanding of the patient, both in terms of realizing their full human potential and also becoming aware of the difficulties and defects which hinder their progress. Ortega's ideas were readily accepted by many homeopaths who felt they could easily categorize their patients' constitutions into one of the three miasmatic concepts.

A few years later, George Vithoulkas proposed that homeopaths don't need to feel limited to three miasms, but that it was possible to consider that tuberculosis could be the origins of the Tubercular miasm in its own right, instead of being the combination of Sycosis and Syphilis as it had been suggested by some authors (H.C. Allen, among others). He proposed a more advanced definition of miasms as "a predisposition to chronic disease underlying the acute manifestations of illness."

But the theory of miasms still remained very obscure. There was no clear idea of what a miasm really was. No thorough understanding of its pattern of manifestation over time, or signs of its recession through a homeopathic healing would be. Decades would pass until the next breakthroughs came forth.

In the later decades of the 20th century a new movement of ideas on health and healing arose and a myriad of books on the meaning of life and the mind/body connection hit the bookshelves. Most of this so called 'New Age' thought was seemingly unrelated to homeopathy, but it ended up becoming a revolution in the way the culture looked at disease and cure. This shift in attitude regarding the meaning of health also eventually shifted the scope of homeopathy and very particularly the theory of miasms.

The new ideas of health and disease looked upon life as a process of evolution. The human being, and therefore health, was no longer considered a static entity which had to preserve a state of innocence or goodness, or a state of strong unpolluted health. The human being was on a journey of evolution, and health was a necessary vehicle in the accomplishment of that journey. For this reason, wellbeing was essential for attaining the best possible results on that path. This concept resonated totally with Hahnemann's own very revolutionary concept of health for his time. Health is what the human being needs "so that our indwelling, reason-gifted mind can freely employ this living, healthy instrument for the higher purposes of our existence."

Disease was now seen not as the old idea of punishment or divine curse for our human sins, but as instances of challenge in our evolutionary path. Our destiny can be realized by facing disease with awareness in a harmonious and creative way. The process of healing involves not only restoring a previous state of health but actually creating a new stage of life for the patient.

In addition, new age medical thinking presented disease as something that arose from the depths of the human being, the manifestation of our own blockages, our own unresolved conflicts from past stages that we had failed to integrate fully into the present moment, rather than something transferred from exterior sources such as infectious bacteria or viruses. Disease was therefore personal and unique to every one of us and was related to our own destiny, ultimately to our own karma. This deeper insight is where the idea of miasms fits in.

Miasms are those deep rivers of susceptibility that bind with the life force from birth and manifest in our bodies, minds and spirits, creating and attracting events and circumstances, specifically customized to our evolutionary needs. Our actions, expressions or outcomes in life come from our instinctive responses dictated by the miasm. Miasms hint at the potential for various possibilities: whether physical, pathological, the resolution of deep issues, or a successful way of life. Miasms are constantly reaffirming the limitations of existence from a physical, emotional and intellectual angle. It is the effort of reducing the control of miasm on a person's life or its total removal that brings forth health. The free will of the individual is held in check by the miasm until it is removed or reduced so that other options are made available.

Miasms also provide the challenges and sufferings we need to resolve in order to heal deeply and to keep pursuing the higher purposes of our existence. Harry van der Zee in his book "Miasms in Labor" proposes a theory of the role of disease and miasms as a necessary stage in the individuation process of mankind: "Miasms offer us the struggle that help us connect with our invincibility, the darkness that makes us discover the light in our soul, the destruction that makes us aware of the indestructibility of our eternal being." Our susceptibility or miasm then is one of the fundamentals tools in the process of human growth. Miasms are the shadow-side of the stages in the evolutionary process.

How can these concepts applied theoretically to the miasms help us as homeopaths in our daily practices? For one thing, they remind us that the ultimate aim of homeopathy as a medical science is not to just treat disease, but to help human beings in their evolutionary path. They also give us an insight into what a deeper knowledge of miasmatic theory can do in terms of prognosis and long term management of our patients. The homeopath must look at the chief complaint as revealing the inner imbalance, and the miasm, the real complex massive disturbance lying beneath.

Our patient's life can seem like a series of random and unpredictable events but through the understanding of miasms a complex pattern of symptoms can be recognized and have meaning to the homeopath. A miasmic prescription frees the organism from the first cause of disturbance, the miasm and its particular disease or problem, and balance is restored. If we can look ahead into our patient's future development down the paths of their miasmatic tendency and select remedies that can act deeply and effectively, and have a firm knowledge of the groups and families of remedies that might act within the different stages and levels of miasms, then we will have truly advanced in our medical art.

B. EVOLUTIONARY SUMMARY OF THE MAJOR MIASMS

The journey of mankind started in oneness, the pre-miasmatic phase where everything was in harmony and mankind was innocent and without individuation. Psora belongs to the phase of separation from this paradise state, where shame, insecurity, nostalgia and hopeful struggle are the themes that predominate. In Sycosis we experience the fixed desperation of our descent into the dark side of our own underworld, which needs to be brought into consciousness. In Syphilis, man struggles to use the amazing powers of creation and destruction that have been awakened in him for the benefit of the whole, instead of for his egotistical needs. From this perspective we need to stop considering miasms as a sequence of stages of decreasing health, and see them as opportunities to affect deep overall healing in the individual.

Each miasm could correspond to a different stage of the life process. Imbalance in higher stages of evolution will have greater consequences; therefore, the corresponding miasm will show deeper states of disease. In homeopathy the Syphilitic remedies tend to be more indicated at the end of life (i.e. heavy metals for neurological diseases of the elderly, like Parkinson's disease), or in younger people with severe degenerative diseases.

The miasm can sometimes be identified by the stage of the disease or type of disease, but it is the larger context of the perception of the patient's experience of his disease that matters. Miasmic prescribing aims to affect more than the disease and return a higher level of freedom, awareness and creativity to the patient.

C. INSIGHT INTO SANKARAN'S MIASMS

In the 1990s Sankaran made a revolutionary step in the understanding and application of miasms. He created a classification and definition of specific miasms that can be recognized in the patient and confirmed through the Vital Sensation. He assigned a specific miasm to individual remedies using a method that is proving to be accurate. He emphasizes that there is one state in a patient that needs to be cured which is discovered by exploring the chief complaint and finding the miasm and the Vital Sensation together. In a cured patient the miasm and the desperation will diminish and will eventually no longer exist.

How to Use Miasms in Casetaking?

The miasm can be seen as a coping mechanism and can be identified by the depth and degree of desperation in the patient. The theme of each miasm represents the way the patient perceives the situation. Someone who needs a Psoric remedy feels that with some struggle it is possible to survive. In a person who needs a Sycotic remedy the problem is irremediable and fixed, and so accepts the situation. In the case of a Syphilitic person there is no hope and they have given up. As one moves from Psoric to Syphilitic, hope decreases and the degree of desperation and sense of isolation increases. The Acute miasm is on the Psoric side of the chart, because there is a lot of hope that the situation is only a temporary threat even though it has the intense desperation of the Syphilitic miasm.

In Dr. Sankaran's analysis there is only one miasm at a given time in a person's life. The patient perceives only one miasm, usually beginning at childhood and does not change that perception, even with changing circumstances. Sometimes the miasm is between two known miasms. For example, a Ringworm case will have signs and language of the Sycotic and Psoric miasms. There is also the possibility that there may be miasms not yet identified at this time, but the miasm is one state throughout the case, even though there may be aspects of other miasms.

The miasm can be identified by the depth and intensity of the perception of the Vital Sensation, a common sensation that connects the mind and the body. For example, the Vital Sensation is of being tied up. A Psoric person can perceive the sensation of tied up as uncomfortable but bearable. A Sycotic person feels he is incapable of freeing himself and so accepts the situation of being tied up. A Tubercular person may feel he is tied up so tightly that it is difficult to breathe. The Syphilic person could be tied up so tightly that there is absolutely no chance of escaping.

The disease state is expressed through the Vital Sensation and the miasm, which the patient experiences as one phenomenon. It is for the sake of selecting a remedy that a differentiation is made between the Vital Sensation and the miasm. The way to distinguish the two separate qualities is by listening for the language of the miasm as the Vital Sensation is probed through the different levels. It is also possible to ask about the miasm, and the Vital Sensation will be expressed. For example, "What is it that you experience so hopelessly?" and the patient replies "I feel hopelessly tied up." There will be many hints of the miasm throughout the case in many of the levels, but it is most reliable when it is expressed with the Vital Sensation.

When the Level of Sensation is reached, the homeopath should observe the Vital Sensation and the miasm together. The miasm is best identified in a case by pursuing the chief complaint until the Vital Sensation is confirmed and then identifying the same miasm at the different levels in the case through the Vital Sensation. At the Level of Fact the intensity of the way the patient is affected and reacts to his chief complaint and local symptoms are indicators of the miasm. At the Level of Emotion, the homeopath can perceive the depth to which the sadness, fear or anger may be felt. At the Level of Delusion, it is possible to see how desperate the patient experiences his false reality. At the Level of Sensation the miasm will be expressed when the Vital Sensation is probed at this level. For example, "How intensely is this sensation experienced?" will often evoke the patient to explain how desperate or hopeful he feels, which will be the miasm.

In order to determine the miasm, often times there is no need to ask a direct question, but to listen to the way the patient presents his chief complaint. When the Vital Sensation is recognized, then see what depth it is experienced. For example the patient might say, "It is as if he hit me so mercilessly and cruelly that there was little chance of survival." Here the Vital Sensation is of someone hitting him, and the depth is mercilessly and cruel with little chance of survival, which indicates the Leprosy miasm.

Questions the homeopath can ask the patient in order to find the miasm:
What is the effect of the chief complaint on you?
How do you perceive your chief complaint or situation?
How do you react to your chief complaint or situation?
How hopeful or desperate do you feel in this situation?

The answers to these questions hint at the miasm. The attitude, actions, and history of the patient can also show the miasm. For example, a patient who tries homeopathy as his last resort is usually very desperate. Another patient who avoids situations, where his asthma may be triggered is adopting an attitude of avoidance (Sycotic miasm). The patient may say that he feels hindered by his disease, which indicates the Malarial miasm, or it feels like a sudden intense violent threat (Acute miasm), or as a critical short lived threatening situation (Typhoid miasm). He may say he hides and covers up the problem (Sycotic miasm), or that he feels hopeless and destructive (Syphilitic miasm). Or he may feel hopeful at times, and at other times acceptance (Ringworm miasm), or feels desperate with very little hope of succeeding (Cancer miasm). A more childlike patient could indicate the Acute or Typhoid miasm, or a more controlling attitude might be the Cancer miasm, etc.

The homeopath can also look at the pace of the case. Is there a sudden rapid phase indicating the Acute miasm? Are there alternating states indicating the Ringworm miasm? Is it more intermittent like the Malarial miasm? These observations are only suggestions of the possible miasm. The best way to confirm the miasm is to understand the patient's experience of the Vital Sensation throughout the case and the different levels by exploring the chief complaint.

The pathology is only a partial expression of the disease state and does not determine the miasm. In some cases the pathology may correspond to the miasm but it is not the sole criterion to determine it. For example a person with pneumonia may need a remedy of the Tubercular miasm if he experiences the Vital Sensation as a feeling of being trapped and needing to get free. Another person may need an Acute miasm remedy, because he experiences the pneumonia as if he will suddenly die and clings to those closest to him. The pathology can be a confirmation of the miasm if the patient confirms the miasm in the Vital Sensation, but in no way should the homeopath automatically determine the miasm based on the pathology.

The Vital Sensation indicates the kingdom, the miasm and the specific sensation of the remedy. For example, if a person feels caught and suffocated, "caught" is the Vital Sensation which may indicate the animal kingdom and "suffocate" represents the Tubercular miasm. Another example is if a person feels so unsupported that they have no one to depend on, and can no longer function. Their whole structure feels as if it has collapsed and is destroyed. The issue of dependence indicates the mineral kingdom and the degree of isolation and destruction is the Syphilitic miasm.

Be aware that the use of certain key words by the patient does not necessarily indicate the miasm. For example, if a patient uses the word "control" does not mean the patient is in the Cancer miasm. The miasm is the depth to which the Vital Sensation is experienced throughout the case. In a Cancer miasm case the Vital Sensation will be experienced as extremely difficult and will require a superhuman effort and control to overcome, not just the fact that the patient used the word "control" to describe his experience.

To avoid confusion between miasms one should refrain from forming quick conclusions. The patient may express the feeling of one miasm, like feeling unfortunate as in the Malarial miasm, and rather than decide the miasm on the basis of this one word, the physician should wait to ascertain the depth and degree of desperation in the case. Those, together with the attitude and other expressions, will clarify the miasm beyond a doubt.

Plant remedies from the same family, or mineral remedies close to each other in the Periodic Table, may have the same or similar sensations, but the depth to which that sensation is experienced or the miasm may be different. Remedies from the animal sub-kingdom often share the same miasm. For example, insect remedies are often but not always Tubercular but not necessarily.

The Vital Sensation of a mineral case will be expressed around issues of structure, which will be more non-human specific (i.e., pressure, heavy, balanced, etc.). The miasm is how the patient views and experiences his issues of structure. A patient, who has a Vital Sensation that the structure does not exist at all, will experience tremendous anxiety, but the situation is not hopeless (Acute miasm possibly Hydrogen). Another patient feels that the structure was built after a lot of effort and now will do everything in his capacity to protect it (Cancer miasm possibly Arsenicum album).

The use of miasms in plant families helps to find accurate remedies by identifying the Vital Sensation in the case and finding the same or a similar sensation in a plant family and then applying the miasm indicated to the selection of the remedy. For example, if the Vital

Sensation in a case is sensitivity and reactivity (plant kingdom) to the sensation of heaviness and floating (Hamamelidae family), which feels nagging and unfortunate (Malarial miasm), the patient may require Cannabis-sativa (a Malarial remedy of the Hamamelidae family). The charts are available in the appendix. But it is important to try to understand the remedies themselves, and not just go from the chart to the prescription, which many people do when first learning this method.

How to Differentiate the Miasm from the Sensation?

It can be difficult to differentiate the miasm from the sensation, especially in plant cases. The forced out sensation of the Liliiflorae family could be confused with the cast out theme of the Leprosy miasm. The patient has the sensation of being suffocated. Is this the Vital Sensation of the Rosacea family or the Tubercular miasm? The homeopath has to find out how is the sensation experienced. The patient says that the sensation of being suffocated feels hopeful and that they can try to overcome it, then the sensation of suffocation is the plant family, and hopefulness and trying is the Ringworm miasm. The remedy to prescribe could be Amygdalus communis (the Ringworm remedy of the Rosaceae family). If the patient says that they feel suffocated in all areas of their life, then the homeopath has to ask how they feel suffocated and the patient may answer that it feels like cutting, stabbing, pinching, etc. (Ranunculaceae family). Then the suffocated sensation indicates the Tubercular miasm and the patient could need Cimicifuga (the Tubercular remedy of the Ranunculaceae family). If the patient expresses over and over the language of the miasm and no other sensation is expressed then the homeopath has to consider the nosode of that miasm. In this example it might be Tuberculinum.

A major discovery was made when plant remedies were categorized by the sensations of the plant family and the miasm. With some plant remedies it is possible to hypothesize what the Vital Sensation and miasm might feel like in the patient. For example, Sarsaparilla is a remedy from the Liliiflorae family, which has the feeling of being excluded or pushed out, and is of the Ringworm miasm with the need to keep trying. In theory the Sarsaparilla patient should be trying not to be excluded, which Dr. Sankaran found to be true in two successful cases.

How are Remedies Categorized into Individual Miasms?

Remedies, especially well proven ones, can be understood based on their sensations as well as the miasm associated with them. The understanding of miasm helps in differentiating between remedies that may have similar symptoms. For example, Sulphur and Platina share the symptom egotism. The Sulphur ego is optimistic and not very desperate (Psoric). The Platina ego is very desperate and can lead to suicide or homicide, and altogether feels quite hopeless (Syphilitic).

Dr. Sankaran's classification of remedies by miasms is done by examining a number of criteria:

1.   Is the remedy known to cure the actual disease, infection or main pathology of a particular miasm? A remedy known to have symptoms of tuberculosis might be considered for inclusion in the Tubercular miasm. Abrotanum has tubercular peritonitis (Boericke) so it has been classified a Tubercular remedy of the Compositae family. For polychrests it is not enough that a remedy is known for a particular disease to include it in that miasm. Lachesis and Arsenicum album are remedies for typhoid fever but they do not belong to the Typhoid miasm because the remedies are known for many different infections. For example, if the remedy has warts or benign tumors prominently the remedy might be classified in the Sycotic miasm.

2.   Do the symptoms of the remedy have specific qualities of the miasm, such as acuteness, intermittency, destructiveness, etc.?

3.   What is the focus of the remedy in the mental state? The dreams, delusions and mental symptoms of the remedy are studied to see if there are characteristics of a particular miasm. For example, Hura and Curare are categorized in the Leprosy miasm because the remedies have strong feelings of dirtiness, disgust and contempt, and feel they are abandoned by family or friends.

4.   What are the most characteristic symptoms of the remedy and do they indicate a particular miasm?

The four criteria are examined in each remedy to make an accurate classification of the miasm. A remedy may have qualities of the miasm indicated before and after it. The process of categorizing individual remedies is ongoing and must be confirmed through our homeopathic clinics. Many remedies have not been categorized because there is not enough information to make a clear distinction at this time. There are also many remedies that seem to have qualities of a number of different miasms. There are a number of differing opinions as to how important the miasm is in certain remedies that do not seem easily catalogued.

D. A STUDY OF INDIVIDUAL MIASMS USING THE REPERTORY

A study of the different miasms was conducted by repertorizing well known remedies from each miasm to understand the characteristic symptoms of the particular miasm. For example, Aconite, Belladona, Arnica and Lyssim, remedies of the Acute miasm, produced the following rubrics:

> Speech & voice; voice; lost; injuries to the head, from
> Kidneys; traumatism of
> Female; pain; labor pains; violent
> Mind; anxiety; abortion, with threatening
> Mind; anguish; cardiac
> Mind; anguish; labor; during
> Sleep; sleepiness; delirium, during

These rubrics indicate trauma that is violent, but without long term destructive symptoms. The chart of rubrics of the other miasms is available in the Repertorization of the Miasms in the Appendix.

Acute Miasm

Acute remedies were used by Hahnemann during acute illnesses such as scarlet fever, pneumonia and delirium and then later were found to also be useful in chronic conditions where the sensation of the patient is identical to the sensation of an acutely ill patient. In the Acute miasm the situation is perceived as temporary but life threatening, as in an acute disease; an intense threat of massive proportions, a sudden, great danger to life. The perception here is hope of recovery in the face of the life threatening situation. The attitude is one of panic, an instinctive fight or flight response. Where the sensation is experienced acutely we could see the individual either escaping for safety until the storm passes, or even having a violent response. There could also be the clinging to others out of a feeling of helplessness. The response often appears childlike. In the failed, uncompensated or more advanced state the person can only act by either panicking, being shocked, stupefied or immobilized.

When the miasm is Acute the person perceives his situation with the same panic as one would experience if they received the sudden news that a bomb was going to go off or if suddenly the ground began to give way beneath their feet. Both situations are life threatening and the state is one of alarm. One's feelings about oneself are not in the forefront. The immediate thing on the person's mind is to save themselves and to flee from danger. In such a situation the person reacts instinctively; or just breaks down out of fear and panic and is unable to do anything. The feeling with such persons is that once they are out of this seemingly threatening situation they will be safe again.

The acute, instinctive response may be mistaken for the desperation of the Syphilitic miasm. Both miasms can be characterized by violence. However, the Acute experience is sudden and the response is instinctive and childish with clinging. The Syphilitic experience on the other hand is permanent, much more destructive and there is complete isolation.

Pathology:
(It is important to note that a person could be in an acute situation or pathology, and experience it with the perception of some other miasm—in which case the appropriate remedy to give would be from that miasm. The Pathology only hints to the miasm.)

Pathology typical to the Acute miasm could include symptoms of extreme intensity that appear and disappear suddenly. Some examples are panic attacks, fevers, asthma, apoplexy, mania.

Veratrum Album – An Acute Remedy:
Veratrum album is one of the well-known Acute remedies. From the Materia Medica we have the following description and symptoms:

Effects are sudden and violent (Phatak)
Fear of death
Ailments from fright
Beside oneself, being
Cut, mutilate, slit, desire to: others
Destructiveness
Escape, attempts to, springs up suddenly
Fear, alone of, being
Shrieking, screaming, shouting: wild, with disposition to bite and tear

From the above symptoms one sees a very acute state. Veratrum album belongs to the plant family Liliflorae, and the common sensation that runs through this family is that of being forced out and excluded, or being oppressed, constrained and constricted; at the level of the mind this sensation is expressed through the feeling of being excluded or left out. This is apparent in the following symptoms:
Despair of social position
Delusion, great person he is
Delusion, squanders money
Loquacity
Lewdness
Singing
Dancing
Kisses everyone
Liar
Deceitful

We can see from these symptoms that there is much concern about his social position, and the loss of it creates despair. He feels okay when he is a great person, a person of some standing. Through other symptoms we can see the attempt to attract attention. The whole of the Veratrum album state is of a man who has suddenly lost his social position, of a king who has suddenly become a pauper. There is a need to regain this position as soon as possible as is apparent from the reactions. At the Level of Sensation the Veratrum album disease can be summed up as forced out or extruded suddenly. The sensation is apparent in the following physical symptoms of the remedy:

Congestion of blood internally

Pain, constricting, orifices, sphincter spasm

Anguish, breathing, with tightness of, oppression, desire to sit up or jump about

The sensation is that of an internal fullness with oppression, constriction and being forced outward. The miasm is Acute.

SUMMARY OF ACUTE MIASM

Sensation:
Sudden great danger
Acute intense threat
Violent threat to life

Success:
Escape
Instinctive action
Besides oneself

Failure:
Panic
Shocked
Stupefied
Immobile

Reaction: Violent, instinctive, strong, urgent
Depth & Degree of Desperation: Acute, critical, Do or Die!
Pace: Sudden, rapid, violent
Pattern: Comes suddenly, lasts a short time, ends suddenly, either in death or recovery
Attitude of the patient: Childlike, instinctive, violent

Age: Infancy
Game: Peek a boo, thrown up in the air and caught
Attitude: Helpless, run for your life, once the danger is passed you are fine again
Picture: Bomb explodes, earthquake

Keywords:
Acute, Sudden, Violent, Panic, Danger, Reflex (action), Escape, Helpless, Terror, Insanity, Infant, Fright, Alarm, Storm, Instinctive (reaction).

Remedies:
Aconite. Arnica. Belladonna. Cactina. Calendula. Camphora. Chocolate. Coffeinum. Croton Tiglium. Digitoxin. Elaterium. Ergotaminum. Hydrogen. Hypericum. Lithium. Melilotus. Morphinum. Oenanthus. Stramonium. Strychninum. Veratrum.
Nosode: Lysinum. Morbillinum. Diptherium.

Typhoid Miasm

This miasm is also known as the Sub-acute miasm. Remedies in this miasm were originally used for typhoid fever, a high, unremitting fever often associated with prostration from violent diarrheas or other infections. The infections are slightly less rapid in their onset (for example Bryonia) than the remedies in the Acute miasm.

The patient feels he is in an urgent, life-threatening situation requiring his full capacity to survive. He is willing to use any means to return to a secure position: violence, scheming, escaping, lying, etc. Willful children who make demands so strongly that their parents' cannot say no often require remedies from this group. The patient's goal is to conserve every resource to combat the threat so there may be themes of preserving business and material needs. The feeling is, "If I can just get through this crisis, I made it and can rest."

The perception is of something sudden, temporary and fatal as in the Acute miasm, however, there is not the instinctive response but a concentrated effort similar to the Psoric miasm. In the Typhoid miasm it is an intense struggle over a short duration. In the successful state the action is a focused effort with impatience, grabbing, do-or-die attitude, taking risks and recovering lost ground. The aim is to come out of a difficult situation as quickly as possible and reach a safe haven and total recovery. In the failed state the effort proves to be excessive, too much activity, which then results in collapse, no more struggling or action.

An example of the Typhoid miasm can be the reaction to a stock market crash. It is a sudden, unexpected, massive and overwhelming event. The person can lose everything and be completely ruined in one stroke. If he struggles and works very hard for a few years after such a loss he might regain his assets and reach his position of security again. The perception here is that if he can make it out of the crisis all is fine, but if he cannot he will be ruined.

The age of the Typhoid miasm is that of childhood. A child of three or four will throw a tantrum when he is refused something. He will demand an object and want it immediately; as soon as it is given to him he will once again be quiet.

The crisis and urgency of the Typhoid miasm may be confused for the hectic pace of the Tubercular miasm and both may appear burnt out in the failed state. The depth and intensity are very different. In the Tubercular miasm the sensation is experienced as oppressive and nearly destructive. Often the patient will use terms like "suffocated" or "trapped" to describe the intensity. The action will be violent and with a desperate attempt to escape, to break free, to change. In the Typhoid miasm the depth is of something sudden, temporary and life threatening. There is a lot of hope, as opposed to the hopelessness of the Tubercular miasm. Also there is an instinctive response with effort in the Typhoid miasm, which may be seen as childish, whereas with the Tubercular miasm there is hopelessness and isolation.

Pathology:
Typhoid remedies can be useful in a variety of chronic conditions such as colitis, Crohn's disease, collapse states, psychosis and psychotic breaks.

Nux Vomica – A Typhoid Remedy:
Nux vomica is a member of the Loganiaceae family, and the sensation is that of being shocked and shattered.

The following rubrics are suggestive of the acuteness of Nux vomica:
Anger, so that he could have stabbed anyone
Beside oneself, being
Break things, desire to
Delusions; imaginations dies; about to, he is
Escape attempts to, springs up suddenly from the bed
Fear driving him from place to place
Fear, panic attacks, empowering

Some other symptoms convey an impression of criticality:
Hurry, haste
Restlessness, nervousness, ardent
Restlessness, nervousness, zealous
Industrious, mania for work

From these symptoms we can see that his reaction to stress is as though the situation is very critical and he needs to make a lot of effort to get over it quickly. Let us now examine what causes stress:
Delusions; imaginations; bed; evening, someone would get into and no room in it, or as if someone has sold it
Delusions; imaginations; bed; someone; in with him
Rest, desire for
Quiet disposition; desires repose and tranquility
Ailments from shock

It is evident that he perceives that his place of rest has been taken away and this is experienced as a shock. His reactions are impulsive and violent as if he was facing something acute, but at the same time he is industrious, ardent, hurried and tries to get back his place of comfort as soon as possible. Once that critical situation has been surmounted, he can rest.

SUMMARY OF TYPHOID MIASM

Sensation:
Bed is sinking
Losing the position of comfort
Sudden loss, business failure
Critical period
Dangerous, risky, urgency
Short lived
Life threatening situation

Success:
Intense short effort
Do or die
Impatience, demanding, taking chances,
Recovering lost ground
Reaching position of comfort
Grab it, want it all, right now!

Failure:
Collapsed
Inactive, given up the struggle, sinking
No effort
No action of the will

Reaction: Concentrated effort and struggle
Depth & Degree of Desperation: Acute, hopeful if concentrated effort is put in. But it is still critical and life threatening.
Pace: Sudden, intense
Pattern: Concentrated effort followed by rest
Attitude of the patient: Childlike

Age: Childhood (1 to 12 years)
Game: Hide and seek
Attitude: If you somehow come out of the crisis all is fine, if you don't you are sunk. Intense short effort needed to find rest.
Picture: House on fire, crash in the stock market

Keywords:
Crisis, Intense, Sinking, Recover, Child, Intense short effort, Typhoid, Sub-acute, Emergency, Homesick, Intense struggle, Critical period, Collapse, Reaching position of comfort, Impatience, Demanding, Right now.

Remedies:
Abelmoschus. Acetic acid. Aethusa. Ailanthus. Anantherum. Argemon. Asclepias tuberosa. Baptisia. Benzoic acid. Bryonia. Carbo animalis. Carbo vegetabilis. Carnegia gigantea. Chamomilla. Doryphora. Euphrasia. Gallic acid. Gambogia. Helleborus. Hyoscyamus. Ipecac. Lycopus. Mancinella. Nux moschata. Nux vomica. Paris quadrifolia. Petroleum. Polystyrene. Podophyllum. Rheum palmatum. Rhus toxicodendron. Sacchrum album. Sulphuricum acidum. Thyroidinum. Veratrum veride. Viscum.
Nosode: Typhoidinum. Pyrogenium.

Psoric Miasm

In the Psoric miasm the depth of perception is much deeper than in the Acute miasm, because the sensation is experienced as permanent. He must struggle against an external problem but is optimistic that he will recover and maintain his position. There is anxiety with doubts about his ability, but he is hopeful and failure does not mean the end of the world.

An example of a Psoric situation is a teenager learning to drive. In the beginning he has a lot of anxiety about his ability, but with some struggle and practice he is able to do it. If he fails there is despair but it is not hopeless, because he has many more opportunities for success ahead.

At this time Lycopodium is the only plant remedy identified in the Psoric miasm. Many of the plant remedies have been reclassified in the Typhoid, Ringworm and Malarial miasms.

Pathology:
Functional pathologies, such as alopecia, vitiligo, etc.

Sulphur – A Psoric Remedy
We can understand Psora through the example of Sulphur, well known to homeopaths as 'the king of anti-psoric remedies.'

Sulphur is a mineral remedy. Sulphur's main problem has to do with structure related to identity (third row in the Periodic Table). The following symptoms exemplify the stress and anxiety of this remedy:
Delusions, he is disgraced
Ailments from embarrassment
Ailments from loss of reputation
Ailments from being scorned

Scorn creates stress in Sulphur, as does being disgraced, or losing their reputation. The depth of reaction to that stress is what classifies him into the Psoric miasm:
Ambition much, ambitious
Business, talks of
Industrious, mania for work

These symptoms show that his action lies in the direction of doing business and making money. Understanding the aim in his ambition and industry will give us a sense of the depth of the turmoil created by the scorn and disgrace.

Other symptoms of Sulphur are:
Delusion, abundance of everything, she has an
Censorious, critical
Egotism, self esteem
Delusions, great person is
Delusions, wealth of

Sulphur's aim seems to be reaching a position where he has more than enough wealth. Then he feels he is great and can criticize others rather than be criticized. He doesn't aim to be the richest person in the world, but just to have more than enough for himself. The aim is not very high; it is well within his reach. The situation is stressful enough to create doubt, but he is also hopeful.

SUMMARY OF PSORIC MIASM

Sensation:
The situation is difficult
The problem is solvable
Optimism
Effort is needed, but it is within my capacity

Success:
Making the effort
Getting it done

Failure:
Gives up hope
Sitting inactively
No more tries

Reaction: Struggle and effort to maintain or recover position
Depth & Degree of Desperation: Very hopeful
Pace: NA
Pattern: Continuous struggle
Attitude of the patient: Hopeful and he must struggle to maintain position

Age: Teenage
Game: Skateboarding
Attitude: If I make an effort, I can do it
Picture: A teenager learning to drive

Keywords:
Struggle, effort, confidence, difficult, hope, anxiety.

Remedies:
Calcarea. Cuprum. Ferrum. Graphites. Kali-Carbonicum. Lycopodium. Niccolum. Sulphur. Zincum.
Nosode: Psorinum

Malarial Miasm

The Malarial miasm lies between the Acute and Sycotic miasms. This miasm is characterized by sudden, acute manifestations that come up from time to time, followed by periods of quiescence. The person perceives an acute threat coming up intermittently in a situation which cannot be changed because of a fixed feeling of deficiency. In the Malarial miasm the feeling is being stuck, hindered, unfortunate and not allowed to come up from the position he is in, since he is regularly tormented by an acute situation of threat. There is also a feeling of powerlessness and dependence.

A typical Malarial situation is someone with an angry boss, who reprimands him from time to time for no apparent reason. The worker cannot retaliate since he is in a helpless and dependent situation. He feels unfortunate that he is stuck in this position where it is impossible to react the way he would like to. All he can do is suppress his anger and fantasize about what he would do to his boss. The only hope in his case is reflected through fantasies rather than any possible real action. In reality, he has no choice but to accept his unfortunate position and suffer the occasional acute torments from his boss.

In the stage of success there is an acceptance of the situation, but from time to time there is also the tendency to get excited and angry. In the stage of failure there is a reaction to the inner feeling of incapability by lamenting, feeling that nothing is good enough, brooding, fantasizing, and having bouts of fears. Malarial is characterized by intermittent acute excitement and acceptance.

Dr. Roger Morrison wrote:

> In Malarial, the situation is still less severe. The patient is suffering but not in imminent danger for his life. Instead he finds himself repeatedly accosted by highly uncomfortable conditions. These conditions leave him weak and vulnerable between the attacks. He is partially crippled by the condition causing him to be dependent on those around him. His forward progress is arrested as he deals with these harassing attacks. For chronic conditions, the remedies of the Malarial miasm feel they are facing recurring attacks from life - they feel stuck in a situation where nothing goes right and he is never truly well. He can do little more than complain or act out. Patients in this miasm often feel miserable and make those around them miserable from their negative outlook.

Roger Morrison points out that the Malaria miasm can easily be confused with the leprosy miasm, because they share the feeling of being unfortunate.

In the malarial miasm, this hopelessness is because of being unable to go ahead, even unable to act on that hopelessness. Morrison cites the rubric *Suicidal disposition, but lacks courage* which appears in China, the main remedy of the Malaria miasm.

As we will see, however, the Leprosy miasm contains elements of social hopelessness not present in the Malaria miasm, the shunned, cast-off feeling of a leper, and a sense of dirtiness and disgust.

Pathology:
Typical pathology would be symptoms with periodic attacks such as: migraine, neuralgia, worms, colic, rheumatism, intermittent fevers, recurring hemorrhoids, recurring or allergic asthma, Meniere's disease, worms, colitis.

Colocynthis – A Malarial Remedy:
If we take Colocynthis as an example of the Malarial miasm we see that the main sensitivity of its plant family, the Violales, is being disturbed. This is expressed through the physical sensations of cutting, lancinating, stitching, sharp, pinching, and the emotional symptoms of vexation, chagrin and being disturbed. If we study the Materia Medica of this remedy, we find lancinating and cutting pains in various parts of the body, especially in the abdomen. There are also the following symptoms:

Vexation; colic causes
Bad effects of vexation
Dreams, vexations
Ailments from mortification, humiliation, chagrin
Disturbed, aversion to being
Pain, neuralgic, intermittent
Abdomen, griping, intermittent, stool after
Violent, periodical or intermittent headache

In fact, many of the complaints, especially the pains, in the scope of this remedy are of an intermittent nature. Some more mental symptoms are:
Escape, attempts to, fever during (acute, instinctive response)
Complaining bitterly day and night
Discontented, displeased, dissatisfied with everything
Greatly affected by the misfortunes of others

The attitude reflected in these symptoms is one of discontentment and complaining. There is an emotional sensitivity to misfortune; this indicates his own sensitivity: he feels unfortunate and unhappy so he complains. All these symptoms indicate the Malarial miasm.

At the deepest level one would expect from the sensation and miasm that the patient experiences his disease as 'intermittently disturbed' or 'persecuted by the disturbance'. This is reflected in the following symptoms:
Agitation; abdomen, with each paroxysm of pain, in
Colic like, spasmodic pain, after vexation
Sharp, spasmodic attacks of pain shooting down the sciatic nerve to the feet
Periodical attacks of fearful, cutting pain in the abdomen

SUMMARY OF MALARIAL MIASM

Sensation:
Stuck and intermittently attacked
Limited
Unfortunate
Imprisoned
Dependent
Fixed weakness within himself that obstructs or hinders
Subject to acute threat or attack to his life

Success:
Accepting his limits; not fighting with them
Intermittent anger
Paroxysms of rage

Failure:
Lamenting, Brooding

Nothing is good
Miserable, Frustration, Discontent
Phobic, paroxysmal fears
Sentimental, Homesick

Reaction: Acceptance of his condition and day dreaming
Depth & Degree of Desperation: An underlying chronic, fixed condition with intermittent acute manifestations
Pace: NA
Pattern: Sudden, acute manifestations which come up from time to time followed by periods of quiescence
Attitude of the patient: Unfortunate, stuck, hindered obstructed and from time to time subject to acute attacks. He can do nothing but accept the situation and daydream.

Age: Childhood to middle age
Game: Blind man's bluff
Attitude: You have to bear it because you are limited therefore dependent.
Picture: Person dependent on his job with an abusive boss (Cinderella complex)

Keywords:
Obstacle, Stuck, Intermittent attack, Persecution, Unfortunate, Paroxysmal, Contemptuous, Disobedient, Periodicity, Harassed, Hindered, Obstructed, Alternation between excitement and acceptance, Torture, Hampered.

Remedies:
Ammonium muriaticum. Angustura. Antimonium crudum. Aurum muriaticum Kalinatum. Berberis. Boletus. Cactus. Capsicum. Cedron. Chelidonium. China (various China salts). Cina. Clematis. Colchicum. Colocynthis. Eupatorium perfoliatum. Eupatorium purpureum. Iris. Kalmia. Magnesia muriatica. Menyanthes. Natrum muriaticum. Peonia. Prunus. Ranunculus bulbosus. Sarracenia. Spigelia. Sumbulus. Verbascum.

Ringworm Miasm

The Ringworm miasm is between Psora and Sycosis, with the characteristics of Psora (the struggle with anxiety about success), as well as characteristics of Sycosis (the fixity resulting from a feeling of inadequacy within oneself). In Ringworm, although there is hope, there is a lot of doubt, much more than in Psora, which is the contribution of the Sycotic component. Ringworm is an infection characterized by phases of intense itching compelling one to scratch; at other times although it is still there it is relatively dormant. Thus there are both, the resigned acceptance as well as the element of struggle. It is an infection which is not life threatening but has the intense struggle at some times but at other times is quiet and fixed, with periods of despair and giving up.

In the proving of the Ringworm nosode, there are dreams and feelings which showed periods of trying with a feeling of hope, and other times there was resignation and acceptance of the situation, only to be followed by another trial.

The situation of the Ringworm miasm seems to be one at the borderline of the person's capacity. There is a struggle with the hope of a possible success and so there is a lot of effort, but each failure makes him give up and accept his limitations. There is alternation between optimism and pessimism. He must continue to try so there is often a cheerful quality and yet he never quite gets there.

This is like an obese person trying to lose weight. There are periods which he really struggles with jogging, walking, exercise and dieting without too much success, and then the feeling that he won't be able to do it and so he gives up and goes back to binging. After a while he renews his struggle and again when nothing happens he gives up. In the active or successful stages he tries and in the failed stages he gives up and is despairing.

Pathology:
Recurrent, non-life threatening illnesses such as Ringworm, tinea, acne, herpetic conditions.

Calcarea Sulphuricum – A Ringworm Remedy:
Calcarea sulphuricum, a salt, contains Calcium (Fourth row in Periodic Table) and Sulphur (Third row). Salts usually have issues of "relationship" as a Vital Sensation. In Calcarea sulphuricum there is a lack of identity (Sulphur) in the place of his security (Calcarea). Identity and security both provide structure for him, and a relationship that provides both would complete the structure.

The need for security is in the following symptoms:
Fear of dark
Fear of night
Timidity

The need for identity is expressed in a desire for appreciation. Calcarea sulphuricum has the single symptom:
Lamenting that he is not appreciated.

His attitude can be understood through the following symptoms:
Quarrelsome
Lamenting
Jealousy
Obstinate
Aversion to persons who do not agree with him
Sits and meditates

A Calcarea sulphuricum person can be obstinate, quarrelsome, complaining (the Ringworm infection itself is fixed and irritating), and at the same time become averse to people who do not appreciate or agree with him. In this way he alternates between complaining and quarreling, and accepting the situation. They can make a lot of effort to be appreciated through their work, manners, appearance, etc.

SUMMARY OF RINGWORM MIASM

Sensation:
Doubts about success
A difficult situation
Not easy
Beyond easy reach

Success:
Alternating between struggle and resignation
Trying

Failure:
Gives up hope
Sitting inactively
No more tries

Reaction: Alternation between acceptance and cover up, hiding, secrecy, unsuccessful efforts, alternation between struggle and giving up
Depth & Degree of desperation: Hope alternating with giving up. Yet it is not fatal and he can live with it.
Pace: NA
Pattern: Periods of effort alternating with periods of inactivity
Attitude of the patient: Sometimes the task seems possible and he is hopeful and struggles to overcome it. Then after awhile he feels that he is inadequate and will not succeed. So he gives up.

Age: Mid twenties to mid thirties
Game: Snakes and ladders
Attitude: I shall try, if I succeed it is good, if I fail I just remain stuck where I am.
Picture: A man, who afraid of water, wants to learn to swim. A 30 year old woman wants to lose weight.

Keywords:
Trying, Giving up, Accepting alternating with trying, Accepting alternating with effort, Irritation, Discomfort, Teenage.

Remedies:
Actea spicata. Allium sativa. Calcarea fluorica. Calcarea silicata. Calcarea sulphurica. Dulcamara. Fagus. Gossypium. Magnesia sulphuric. Opunta vulgaris. Pseudotsuga. Rhus senanata. Sarsaparilla. Taraxicum. Teucreum. Upas. Veronica officianalis. Viola tricolorata. Lac humanum. Gorilla's milk.
Nosode: Ringworm nosode.

Sycotic Miasm

The sensation here is experienced to a depth that makes it appear permanent and fixed but not destructive. With the Psoric miasm there is hope and a corresponding attitude of struggle. In a Sycotic case, the sensation is that something is fixed and irremediable, so hope is replaced by acceptance.

The Sycotic attitude is to accept, avoid, hide and cover up a situation they cannot deal with. Such attitude comes after a long unsuccessful struggle with the problem. The person gives up the struggle feeling he lacks the capacity to do anything about the situation; so he accepts it but makes sure his incapacity is hidden from others. With the admission of his inner weakness there is an attempt to cope by secrecy, egotism and compulsive acts. Therefore the Sycotic person is closed because he has something to hide. He will not relate openly to others; his interaction is limited to a few trusted people. There are also many fixed ideas, ritualistic and compulsive acts. In the failed states there is guilt, remorse, self-reproach and a feeling of exposure.

Sycotic tendencies are typical of middle age; it also lies in the middle of the miasmic chart. This is the time when ideas become rigid, personal freedom is restricted and the person is content to accept rather than struggle. One can see that such a feeling of having to accept and live with a circumstance would arise after having struggled in vain for a long time. Thus it is possible to see that Psora is the mother of the Sycotic miasm. With the Psoric miasm there is hope and a corresponding attitude of struggle. In a Sycotic case, hope is replaced by acceptance.

Dr. Roger Morrison describes the correlation between the Sycotic miasm and the sexually transmitted disease it is named after:

> *Gonorrhea is a condition that is not life-threatening but is shameful and embarrassing. The remedies used to combat gonorrhea and gleet also treat the ailments of suppressed gonorrhea. All of the diseases that respond to this group of remedies are fixed and intractable: They do not go away but they do not progress. The patient spends a great deal of time trying to cover up or compensate for the illness. Thus we have the well-known characteristic of the Sycotic miasm: secretiveness. The patient is often riddled with guilt and insecurity. Inferiority complex is a common finding in this miasm.*

Pathology:
Typical pathology of the Sycotic miasm is: asthma, neuroses, warts, growths, physical conditions often center around the urinary or genital tract, tumors and neoplasms, eczema, genital herpes.

Thuja – A Sycotic Remedy:
Thuja is one of the main remedies in the Sycotic miasm. This is a plant remedy in the Conifer family. The main sensations of the Coniferea are fragile, broken, brittle, disconnected, fragmented, cut off. These sensations are evident in the following symptoms:
Delusions, imaginations, body; brittle is
Delusions, imaginations; body; delicate
Delusions, imaginations; thin; body is

Delusions, imaginations; body parts, continuity of will dissolve
Delusions, imaginations; glass, she is made of

The degree of desperation and attitude can be seen through some other symptoms:
Fanaticism
Monomania

These symptoms convey the impression of fixedness in actions and attitude. Some more symptoms are:
Insanity, madness; touched, will not be
Fear; approaching; others, of
Fear; struck by those coming toward him, of being

What is apparent here is a fixed feeling of fragility and brittleness and the corresponding action of not allowing anyone to touch or approach him, avoiding in this way to be broken. At the level of sensation the Thuja disease can be summed up as 'covering up for the brittleness.' Thuja patients can be secretive, hiding and covering up this inner sense of fragility; which in emotional terms could be translated as an inner inadequacy.

SUMMARY OF SYCOTIC MIASM

Sensation:
There is a fixed, irremediable weakness within the self, which must be covered up and hidden.

Success:
Keeping the weak spot hidden from the view of others
Fixed ideas and ritualistic behavior
Everything is covered up
Hypersensitive to certain things and so leads a very restricted life

Failure:
Guilt
Remorse
Self-reproach
Being exposed

Reaction: Acceptance. Cover up, hiding, secrecy
Depth & Degree of desperation: It is not fatal, but it is fixed and he will have to accept it and live with it.
Pace: Fixed
Pattern: Fixed
Attitude of the patient: I cannot do anything about it, so I must accept it and live with it. I am okay so long as I am able to cover it up.
Age: 35 to 50
Game: Poker (others shouldn't see your hand)
Attitude: It can't change, and I will not let there be any change

Picture: Person practicing without proper qualifications

Keywords:
Fixed, Covered-up, Guilt, Hide, Secretive, Fixed weakness, Avoidance, Accepting, Middle age.

Remedies:
Argentum metallicum. Borax. Bovista. Calcarea bromata. Cannabis indica. Caulophyllum. Crocus sativa. Digitallis. Gelsemium. Kali bichromicum. Kali bromatum. Kali sulphuricum. Lac caninum. Lac delphinum. Natrum sulphuricum. Palladium. Pulsatilla. Sabadilla. Sanguinaria. Silica. Thuja.
Nosode: Medorrhinum

Cancer Miasm

The Cancer miasm lies between the fixity of the Sycotic miasm and the destruction of the Syphilitic miasm. The sensation is perceived to a depth where it is seen as a chaos which is going out of control into destruction and the person has limited abilities to bring the situation back under control. There is a feeling of weakness and incapacity within, and the need to perform exceedingly well and live up to very high expectations. The reaction is a superhuman effort, stretching himself beyond the limits of his capacity, in order to bring the chaos under control. It is a continuous and prolonged struggle which seems to have no end. His survival depends on it, for failure would mean, death and destruction. Unlike the Syphilitic miasm, the experience is not completely destructive; there is some hope of establishing control.

Dr. Roger Morrison wrote of the correlation between the Cancer miasm and the desperation of the typical cancer patient:

> *When a patient receives a diagnosis of cancer, it is obvious that the condition is life threatening. The patient and the family feel there is almost no hope but yet they do not give up. They search high and low for a new drug trial, a new surgery, or even a farfetched alternative like homeopathy. The feeling is one of desperation, of holding on to hope with the fingernails. The patient who needs a remedy from this miasm feels he must carry out his life perfectly - one failure of duty, one lapse in cleanliness, one cheat of the proper diet and all will be lost. Perfectionism and the need for control with the feeling of being strained to one's very limit are the normal presentation.*

Pathology:
Physically the Cancer miasm is often found in patients with a history of cancer but many other physical ailments can be produced. Anorexia nervosa is often treated by remedies of this miasm. Tumors of any sort, neurological disorders such as multiple sclerosis are often found in this miasm.

Ignatia – A Cancer Remedy:
Ignatia is a Cancer remedy from the Loganiaceae family. The Vital Sensations that runs through remedies of this plant family are: shocked, shattered, torn to pieces, ruined, let down, disappointed. This is evident in the following symptoms:
Delusion, ruined, he is
Ailments from shocks, grief, disappointment
Generalities, torn to pieces, shattered pain as if
Pain: bursting, splitting, driver asunder
Paralysis: mental shock from

The theme of keeping control is seen in the following symptoms:
Ailments from: anger, vexation: grief, with silent
Ailments from: anger, vexation: suppressed
Grief: undemonstrative

The Vital Sensation in Ignatia is: He must keep control during shock and disappointment, which would otherwise shatter him. This sensation is in the symptom:
Grief: silent: love, with disappointed.

SUMMARY OF CANCER MIASM

Sensation:
Task is much beyond my limits
Things are going out of control and it will all be destroyed if I do not succeed in keeping the control
Chaos
Breaking away
Fixed weakness within

Success:
Stretching beyond the limit to keep things in control
Total control on self and surroundings
Perfectionist and fastidious

Failure:
Everything is going out of control and I can do nothing

Reaction: In order to gain control over the chaos he must make a superhuman effort and stretch himself far beyond his limited capacity.
Depth & Degree of Desperation: Desperate with very little hope of succeeding, but it is not altogether hopeless
Pace: Rapid and destructive
Pattern: NA
Attitude of the patient: Trying to gain control over a situation that is far beyond his capacity. Demanding too much of himself. Perfection.

Age: Sixty to seventy

Game: Juggling on a tightrope
Attitude: Small person with a huge task to keep things in total control
Picture: A child of alcoholic parents in which her world is chaotic

Keywords:
Control, Perfection, Fastidious, Beyond one's capacity, Superhuman, Cancer, Great expectation, Chaos, Order, Stretching beyond capacity, Loss of control, Self-control.

Remedies:
Agaricus, Anacardium. Anhalonium, Argentum nitricum, Arsenicum album. Asarum. Baryta arsenicum, Bellis perennis, Calcarea arsenica, Calcarea nitrica, Causticum, Conium. Ferrum Arsenicum, Ignatia, Kali arsenicum, Kali nitricum, Natrum arsenicum, Nitricum acidum, Opium, Physostigma, Ruta, Sabina, Staphysagria, Tabacum, Viola odorata.
Nosode: Carcinosinum, Scirrhinum.

Tubercular Miasm

The Tubercular miasm lies between Sycotic and Syphilitic, where the situation is viewed as oppressive, where one's weakness is being exploited. It is at a greater depth and with more desperation than with the Cancer miasm. There can be feelings of suffocation, being caught or trapped in a situation with no way out, being compressed, the gap narrowing. The reaction is the desire to break free, to get out or to escape. The patient may appear burnt out from the hectic pace, there is very little hope and destruction seems imminent.

In the proving of Bacillinum, many provers had dreams of quick and intense activity, and used the word "hectic" to describe their dreams. Other significant dreams included those of being in a narrow restaurant, feeling oppressed and imprisoned in concentration camps.

The attitude in the Tubercular miasm is that time is too short, and that there is too much to be done in too little time. While in success there is hectic activity and a lot of effort to bring about change or to get out, in failure there is the attempt to break free or burst out with violence and destruction.

Dr. Roger Morrison writes: "The feeling of the miasm relates to the ever encroaching and eventually fatally suffocating infection. The patient rebels, struggles, longs for freedom from his condition. He hurries to live his life even as he intuits that it is burning away from him. He feels the walls closing in upon him. His loved ones cannot be trusted."

Pathology:
A.D.D., tuberculosis, asthma, respiratory conditions, persecution complex, deformative arthritis.

Tarentula Hispanica – A Tubercular Remedy:
Tarentula hispanica is industrious, busy, lots of energy, and has a love for music, dancing and colors. There is also the fear of being assaulted, injured, and of getting trapped. Other prominent features are haste, hurry and impulsiveness, which clearly indicate the Tubercular miasm and are similar to features of the nosode Tuberculinum. Sometimes it is difficult to

differentiate Tarentula hispanica from Tuberculinum in a child who has restless behavior, increased energy and is disobedient. Tarentula also has intense anxiety states, fear of being trapped, and attacks of suffocation with the desire for fresh air.

Symptoms from Phatak are:
Activity, fruitless
Hands restless
Walk, impulse to

SUMMARY OF TUBERCULAR MIASM

Sensation:
Intense oppression; things are closing in or narrowing down and there is a desperate desire for change

Caught and suffocated
Compressed
Gap is narrowing
Time is short

Success:
Hectic activity to get out

Failure:
Burnt out going towards total destruction

Reaction: Intense, hectic activity in order to break free from the oppression
Depth & Degree of Desperation: Desperate with very little hope of breaking free
Pace: Very rapid and destructive
Pattern: NA
Attitude of the patient: There is a radical and violent reaction with hectic activity for him to come out of his intense oppressive feeling.

Age: 60 to 70
Game: "Beat the Clock"
Attitude: Time is short, I have to do so much in this time
Picture: A Jewish person in Nazi Germany just before the war

Keywords:
Hectic, Intense activity, Suffocation, Trapped, Closing in, Change, Activity, Freedom, Defiant, Tuberculosis, Oppression, Desire to change.

Remedies:
Abrotanum. Acalypha. Apis. Aranea. Arsenicum iodatum. Atrax. Balsamum. Brucea. Bromium. Calcarea iodata. Calcarea phosphorica. Cereus bonplandii. Cimicifuga. Cistus. Coccus cacti. Coffea. Drosera. Elaterium. Euonymus. Ferrum iodatum. Ferrum phosphoricum. Fluoric acid. Ginseng. Iodum. Kali phosphoricum. Latrodectus. Magnesia

phosphorica. Mygale. Myristica. Myrtus communis. Natrum phosphricum. Oleander. Phelandrium. Phosphorus. Pix. Rumex. Salix niger. Sambucus. Senega. Succinic acid. Tarentula. Theridion. Ustilago. Verbascum.Vespa.
Nosode: Bacillinum. Tuberculinum (in all its preparations). BCG vaccine.

Leprosy Miasm

The miasm is close to the Syphilitic miasm with nearly the same amount of oppression, destruction, desperation, hopelessness and isolation, but with a desire for a radical change. The difference between the Tubercular and the Leprosy miasm is the feeling of misfortune. Hura, a remedy often used to treat leprosy, has the symptom "excited and oppressed, as if by some misfortune," in Allen's Encyclopedia.

Traditionally, the reaction to people with leprosy has been disgust. Leprosy is a slowly progressive condition that ends in death, and often involves terrible disfiguration. Their family may abandon them and society isolates them in leper colonies. In the leprosy miasm we see the suffering caused by feelings of being shunned for some sort of dirtiness or disgusting condition, along with a sense of hopelessness of ever finding a cure.

A person needing a remedy from the leprosy miasm may feel mocked and criticized by his friends and family. There is also the unfortunate and helpless feeling as if he was cursed. He feels self-contempt and dirty. He may have disgusting dreams showing the depth of the dirty feeling inside. Sometimes these feelings may be reflected in the actions of the patient, in cursing, contempt and disgust for others and shunning them.

He may feel hunted down, pushed into a corner and destroyed. His reaction may be contemptuous and treating others as outcastes, sometimes even imagining he is someone really great, isolating himself in a way that makes it appear as if he is too good to mix with ordinary people. In a failed state he acts by shutting himself up totally, isolating himself with the feeling that he is disgusting and that people despise him, complete despair; in this state there can also be suicidal and homicidal reactions.

Pathology:
Suicidal thoughts or impulses, depression, morbid obesity.

Sepia – A Leprosy Remedy:
Sepia has the Vital Sensation of the animal kingdom, victim versus aggressor, weaker versus the stronger, and the main issue of survival. In Sepia the specific issue is of domination by someone stronger or more powerful than her. Sepia has the symptoms:
Ailments from: domination by others, a long history of
Delusions something comes from above which oppresses the chest
Undertakes things opposed to his intentions.

Sepia patients can also be independent, which is reflected in the symptoms:
Industrious, mania for work
Occupation, ameliorates.

They are sensitive to domination and resent being dominated. By being active and industrious they are able to be independent of the domination. The miasm is evident in the following symptoms:

Anxiety: oppressive
Aversion: husband, to
Company: aversion to, aggravates: avoids the sight of people, lies with closed eyes
Delusions, unfortunate he is
Delusions, alone in a graveyard
Estranged from her family
Suicidal despair from his miserable existence
Discouragement, often to such an extent as to be disgusted with life
Repugnance to customary business
Repugnance and dislike to food.

She has the feeling that she has to do what she does not want to. She is being forced and dominated and not allowed to have her way.

SUMMARY OF LEPROSY MIASM

Sensation:
Hunted down
Isolated
Poisoned
Destroyed
Dirty
Disgusting, despised
Pushed to a corner

Success:
Avoids the sight of people
Contemptuous

Failure:
Suicidal
Homicidal
Tears himself
Bites
Despair

Reaction: Violence, shuts himself up, avoids the sight of people, isolates
Depth & Degree of Desperation: Desperate with very little hope of succeeding
Pace: Very rapid and destructive
Pattern: NA
Attitude of the patient: He is doomed, therefore, he gives up.

Keywords:

Disgust, Great contempt, Isolation, Mutilation, Intense hopelessness, Intense oppression, Dirty, Hunted, Tears himself, Bites, Despair, Outcast, Sadism, Repulsion, Loathing, Confine, Castaway, Seclude.

Remedies:
Agraphis. Aloe. Ambra grisea. Androctonus. Aristolochia. Aurum sulphuricum. Azadirachta. Baryta iodata. Baryta sulphurica. Cereus serpentinus. Cicuta. Coca. Codeinum. Comocladia. Curare. Cyclamen. Fumaria. Gratiola. Homarus. Hura. Hydrastus. Hydrocotyle. Indolum. Iodum. Kola. Laurocerasus. Ledum. Mandragora. Mephites. Ocimum sanctum. Rhus glabra. Secale. Sepia. Skatolum. Solanum tuberosum Aegrotans. Spiraea.
Nosode: Leprominium.

Syphilitic Miasm

The experience of the sensation here is very deep, so much so that is seems permanent, destructive and fatal. The feeling is that he is faced with a situation beyond salvage, leading to complete hopelessness, intense desperation and despair. It is a no way out situation where the highest and sole responsibility rests entirely on one person's shoulders. There is far less chaos, higher stakes and more destruction than in the Cancer miasm. The response to this feeling in the success stage is taking it on, doing the utmost by taking up the highest position as leader or king, taking all responsibility by himself. In the failed stage there may be a desperate effort in which the person tries to change either himself or the situation and the result is usually destruction. The desperation may be seen in a drastic, last ditch, do or die effort, or in extremely violent actions, suicidal or homicidal impulses.

To get an idea of the Syphilitic situation one could think of the captain of a sinking ship. The entire responsibility of saving the lives of many people rests singly upon him—whereas the Cancer miasm might be captain of a ship in which a mutiny is taking place, and he needs to regain control over the chaos. When the situation gets totally out of his control and doom seems inevitable, he can either take on the task far beyond his capacity and do his best, or he may totally give up out of despair since all is lost anyway.

The extreme hopelessness of the Syphilitic patient is also reflected in an intense feeling of isolation. The person cannot change the predicament himself, nor can anyone else help him. In some ways the situation of the Syphilitic miasm may seem similar to the acute miasm, however, since the sense is of being alone to face destruction, one doesn't see the instinctive clinging of the Acute miasm. Often this tremendous sense of isolation is expressed in the feeling of being completely alone in the world.

Syphilitic personalities have a strongly pessimistic view of life. They believe it is impossible to change what has gone wrong; the situation needs to be radically changed or else destroyed. This internal feeling makes them react drastically in the face of any external situation: Their reactions are often violent and destructive towards themselves and others. The Syphilitic person has very rigid ideas, verging on fanaticism.
The age of the Syphilitic miasm is that of senility. There is no hope now, the struggle is over. Even coping with oneself is not possible. The end result is death.

Dr. Roger Morrison writes: "Syphilis was an inexorable death sentence in the pre-antibiotic era. The condition is utterly destructive - either physically or mentally. Extreme nihilism marks the patient in the uncompensated state. The diseases are destructive of bone and tissue leading eventually to death. The patient reacts to his illness or his perceived life situations as though under a death sentence. He is prone to feelings of violence and revenge. Suicide or homicidal feelings are common. Destructive addictions often result."

Pathology:
Cardiac conditions, aortic disease, aneurysm, alcoholism, ulcers, heart attacks, paralysis, psychosis, suicidal depression, destructive addictions.

Alumina – A Syphilitic Remedy
Alumina is a mineral remedy with the main issue of identity. It belongs along with the other third row of the periodic table along with Natrum, Magnesium, Silica, Phosphorus, Sulphur and Chlorum.

In Alumina the main sensation is a complete lack of identity, so that he does not know who he is at all. A complete lack of identity would create tremendous desperation. In some instances, the person takes on the identity of another person, his spouse, father or mother. Without that person the patient would be unable to survive, and on occasions where these relationships were threatened they would attempt suicide. There seems to be a complete destruction of identity. The patient has the feeling as though another person has said or seen what he saw, as though he was placed inside another person and only then could see it. It is the sensation as if his self-consciousness was outside his body.

Among the most well-known symptoms of Alumina are:
Confusion of mind; identity, as to his own, as if it were not his
Delusions, identity, errors of personal
Suicidal disposition; seeing: blood or a knife, she has horrid thoughts of killing herself, although she abhors the idea
Despair; recovery, of

SUMMARY OF SYPHILITIC MIASM

Sensation:
There is no hope and this is far beyond my capacity
The unpardonable crime
He has the highest and sole responsibility
The situation is desperate and beyond salvage and there is no hope of succeeding

Success:
Taking it on, doing the utmost
High position, leader, king
Failure:
Suicidal, complete despair,
Destructive acts, homicide, suicide.
Self destructive like alcoholism,
Catatonic, withdrawn, total indifference

Reaction: Desperate, last ditch effort or despair.
Depth & Degree of desperation: Very deep, great desperation, absolutely no hope of success
Pace: Destructive
Pattern: NA
Attitude of the patient: The situation is completely out of his reach. But he must make a last ditch, desperate attempt to come out of it even though there is no hope of succeeding.

Age: Beyond 80
Game: Playing chess with the computer
Attitude: The task is hopeless, but let me do the best I can.
Picture: The captain of a sinking ship

Keywords:
Destruction, Homicide, Suicide, Ulcers, Total, Impossible, Despair, Psychosis, Devastation

Remedies:
Alumina. Anagallis. Aurum. Cenchris. Clematis. Crataegus Echinacea. Elaps. Hepar sulphur. Hydrocotyle. Lachesis. Lathyrus. Leptandra. Mercurius. Origanum. Osmium. Naja. Platinum Plumbum. Plutonium. Psilocibe. Stillingea. Baryta carb.
Nosode: Syphilinum.

E. APPENDIX

CHARTS

PACE

Acute	Typhoid	Psoric	Sycotic	Malarial
Sudden, rapid, violent	Rapid, sudden, intense		Fixed	Intermittent

Ringworm	Cancer	Tubercular	Leprosy	Syphilitic
Alternating	Rapid, destructive	Very rapid and destructive	Very rapid and destructive	Destructive

PATTERN

Acute	Typhoid	Psoric	Sycotic	Malarial
Comes suddenly, lasts short time, ends suddenly, either in death or recovery	Concen-trated effort followed by rest	Continuous struggle	Fixed	Sudden, acute manifestations which come up from time to time followed by periods of quiescence
Ringworm	Cancer	Tubercular	Leprosy	Syphilitic
Periods of effort alternating which periods of inactivity				

ATTITUDE

Acute	Typhoid	Psoric	Sycotic	Malarial
Childlike, instinctive, violent	Childlike	Hopeful and he must struggle to maintain position	I cannot do anything about it, so I must accept it and live with it. I am okay so long as I am able to cover it up.	Unfortunate, stuck, hindered obstructed and from time to time subject to acute attacks. He can do nothing but accept the situation and day dream

Ringworm	Cancer	Tubercular	Leprosy	Syphilitic
He alternates. Sometimes the task seems possible and he is hopeful and struggles to overcome it. Then after a while he feels that he is inadequate and will not succeed. So he gives up.	Performs to gain control over a situation that is far beyond his capacity. Demanding too much of himself. Perfectionist.	If he has to come out of this intense oppression there must be a change, which may be radical and violent, and for this hectic activity is required.	He is doomed and so he can do nothing about it. He gives up.	The situation is completely out of his reach. But he must make a last ditch, desperate attempt to come out of it even through there is no hope of succeeding.

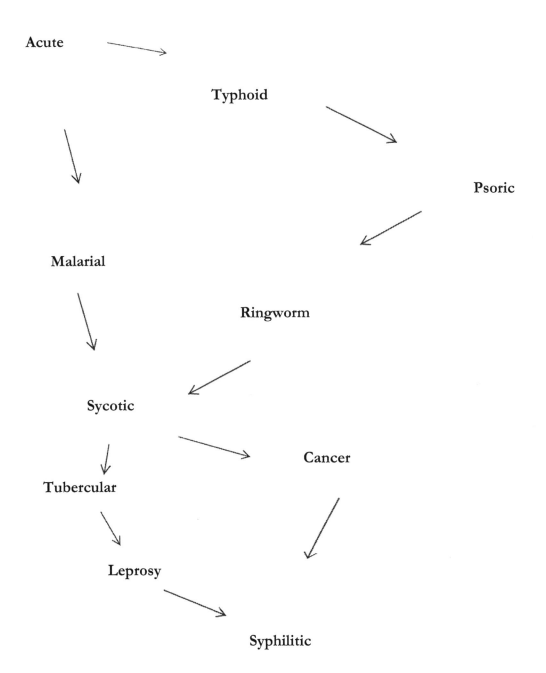

MIASMS	ANIMALS	MINERAL
Acute	Lysinum	Chloralum, hydrogen, lithium
Typhoid		
Psoric		Calc carb, cupr, nat carb, sulph
Sycotic	Lac caninum, moschus	Antim crud, kali brom (near sycotic), calc brom, cobalt, ferrum met, kali carb, mag carb manganum, pallad, polyst, silica, caust
Ringworm	Lac humanum	Calc silic, cal sul, kali sul, mag sul, carb oxygen
Malarial	Lac defloratum, ratus	Ammon carb, ammon mur, chininum salts, china sul, mag mur, nat mur
Turbercular	Apis, tarentula hispanica, theridion, mephites, spiders and insects, spongia	
Cancer	Asterias ruben, elaps corr	Arg-nit, ars alb, calc nit, kali ars, nit-acid, salts of ars
Leprosy	Ambra gr., blata orientalis, Sepia	Adam, kali iod, bary iod, nat iod,
Syphilitic	Bufo, hippomanes Lac leoninum, snakes, scorpion, maias-l	Arg met, aur met, baryta, hepar sulph, osm, plati, plumb, plutonium

MIASMS	Plants
Acute	Acon, Agath-a, arbutinum, arnica, ayahuasca, bell, cactina, calendula, camphor, chocol, coffinum, croton tig, digita, elaterium, hypericum, lepidium, mellotus, morphinum, oenanthe crocata, pyrus americana, stram, strychnine, verat alb
Typhoid	Abelmoschus hib, aethusa, ailanthus, argemone mex, arum-triph, baptisia, bryonia, carnegi gigan, chamom, euphrasia, gaultheria, hyoscyam, ipecac, lycopus, mancin, nux mosc, nux vom, paris quad, podoph, rhus-tox, sinapis-nigr, terebinth, helleborus niger
Psoric	Lycopodium
Sycotic	Asa foetida, caladium, cannabis indica, cauloph, cinnamonium, cochlearia, copiva, crocus sativus, digitalis purp, fabiana imbric, gambogia (ringworm?), gelsemium, helonias, lillium tig, luffa operculata, mangifera indica, piper-nigrum, ptelea, puls, rhod, sabadila, sangunaria, senecioaureus, thuja, tilia, tribulus, yohimbinum

Ringworm	
Malarial	Abies nigra, abroma aug, angustura, arum-ma, berb vulg, cactus grandifl, cann-s, capsicum, casc, chelido majus, chelone glabra, china, china sulph, cina, cochcum autumnale, colocynthis, dioscorea villosa, eupatorium perf, iberis, kalmia, lysimachia numm, myric, ranunc bulb, ranunc scleratus, rhus-radicans, robinia pseud, spigelia, verbas, sumbulus moschatus
Tubercular	Abrotanum, acalypha indica, agraphis nutans, atropinium purum, balsum peruvi, cereus bonplandii, cimicifuga, cistus canad, coffea, guaicum, juglans-ca, myristica, phellandrium aquatic, piper-m, pix liquida, succinic acid, teucriu scoro, thiosina
Cancer	Agnus-c, anac, anha, asarum, bell p, chimaphi, conium, galium asp, ign, opium, ornithog, oxalis, physost, rosemary, ruta, sabina, scrophularia, nodsa, staph, tabacum, ulm, viola odorata
Leprosy	Aloe, arist, caesalp, cast-v, cereus serp, cicuta, coca, cocainum, codeinum, comocladia, cubeba, curare, cyclamen, gratiola, hydrastis can, inula helenium, kola, lactuca vir, lappa, laurocerasus, ledum, mandragora, ocmum sanct, raphanus, rhus glabra, xanthoxylum, thea
Syphilitic	Anagallis, berb-aqu, clematis, corydalis, echinacea, franc, hoang nan, hydrocotyle, jaborandi lathyrus crat, juglans-r, lath, leptan, origanum, stiliangia sylva

MIASMS	NOSODE
Acute	Lysinum, Morbillinum, Diptherium
Typhoid	Pyrogenium, Typhoidinum
Psoric	Psorinum
Malaria	
Ringworm	Ringworm nosode
Sycotic	Medorrhinum
Cancer	Carcinosinum, Scirrhinum
Turbercular	Bacilinum, Tuberculinum, BCG Vaccine
Leprosy	Leprominium
Syphilitic	Syphilinum

Alert words can represent the Vital Sensation or the Miasm. Please check the appropriate box to be analyzed correctly.

Alert words	Represents the Miasm (the pace, the depth, the degree of the Vital Sensation)	Represents the Vital Sensation (kingdom or non-human specific language)	If you are not sure then analyze for both the kingdom and the miasm

Acute Miasm:

Using MacRepertory, a search was made for rubrics containing at least three of four Acute miasm remedies, Acon, Bell, Arn, Lyss. The list was sorted to put the smallest rubrics first:

Speech & voice; voice; lost; injuries to the head, from

Kidneys; traumatism of

Female; pain; labor pains; violent

Mind; anxiety; abortion, with threatening

Mind; anguish; cardiac

Mind; anguish; labor; during

Sleep; sleepiness; delirium, during

Typhoid Miasm:

In MacRepertory, a search was made for rubrics containing at least three of four remedies, Bry, Bapt, Hyos and Rhus-t. The resultant list was then sorted, with the smallest rubrics first. The rubrics noted were:

Fever; Mediterranean fever

Fever; continued fever, typhus, typhoid; soreness, muscular, with

Mind; fear; sold, of being

Fever; continued fever, typhus, typhoid; night; temperature running very high

Fever; continued fever, typhus, typhoid; headache, with

Mind; business; talks of; delirium, during

Mind; delirium; talking, with; business, of

Mind; delirium; busy

Mind; delusions; bed; sinking, were

Fever; continued fever, typhus, typhoid; pneumonia, with; bronchial symptoms

Fever; continued fever, typhus, typhoid; pectoral

Rectum; diarrhea; typhoid fever, from

Mind; dreams; exertion; physical

Mind; bed; get out of, wants to

Mind; escape, attempts to; run away, to

Generalities; change; desire for change of position

Fever; continued fever, typhus, typhoid; cerebral

Mind; anxiety; bed; driving out of

Mind; delusions; home; away from, is

Malarial Miasm:

The MacRepertory search was limited to four remedies, Nat-m, Chin, Caps, Spig. Rubrics containing at least three of the four remedies were selected and then sorted so that the smallest rubrics come first.

Stomach; appetite; ravenous, canine, excessive; worms, from

Head pain; general; Malarial, in

Perspiration; periodical

Similarly, a list containing only two of the four remedies mentioned above:

Respiration; impeded, obstructed; palpitation

Respiration; impeded, obstructed; sticking; epigastrium in

Mind; forgetful; periodical

Mind; memory; weakness, loss of; periodical

Generalities; pulse; intermittent; every; other beat

Chill; anticipating; every; other day; one hour

Ringworm Miasm:

Five remedies were selected for the MacRepertory search, Calc-s, Calc-sil, Viol-t, Dulc, Chrysar. Rubrics containing at least two of these remedies were then selected and sorted with the smallest rubrics coming first.

Extremities; warts; hand; large

Skin; warts; hard

Skin; warts; inflamed

Mind; irritability; daytime

Head; eruptions; tinea; favosa capitis, scaldhead, porrigo, ringworm

Skin; eruptions; herpetic; dry

Skin; eruptions; herpetic; stinging

Skin; eruptions; herpetic; moist

Sycotic Miasm:

Thuja, Sil, Nat-s and Med were selected for the MacRepertory search. Rubrics containing at least three of these remedies were selected and the resultant list was then sorted, with the smallest rubrics first.

Respiration; asthmatic; Sycotic

Bladder; catarrh; gonorrhea, from suppressed

Extremities; callosities, horny; soles, on; tenderness

Skin; warts; soft

Prostate; hardness

Mind; weeping, tearful mood; spoken to, when

Female; menses; staining; fast

External throat; warts

Urethra; discharge; gleety; suppressed

Generalities; discharges; stain indelibly fast

Mind; ailments from; anticipation, foreboding, presentiment; examination, before

Mind; anxiety; anticipating; engagement, an

Mind; washing; always; hands, her

Skin; warts; pedunculated

Mind; fear; examination, before

Skin; moles

Mind; delusions; pursued, he was

Eye; tumors; tarsal tumors

Mind; timidity; public, about appearing in

Female; condylomata

Generalities; tumors, benign

Male; gonorrhea; chronic, sub-acute stage

Mind; introverted

Tubercular Miasm:

Cal-p, Tub, Dros and Phos were selected for the search. Rubrics with at least three of these four remedies were selected and sorted.

Chest; narrow

Mind; anger, irascibility; temper tantrums; attention, to obtain

Female; sexual desire; increased; nursing child, when

Mind; wander; desires to; place to place, from

Mind; nymphomania

Mind; kicks; sleep, in

Cancer Miasm:

Carc, Arg-n, Nit-ac, Con, Ars, Staph and Anac were the remedies selected for the search. Rubrics with at least three remedies were selected and sorted.

Male; excrescences; epithelioma on glans

Mind; jumping; impulse to; height, from a

Mind; rest; cannot, when things are not in proper place

Mind; anger, irascibility; mistakes, over his

Abdomen; liver and region of, ailments of; cancer

Mind; ailments from; rudeness of others

Leprosy Miasm:

A MacRepertory search was made for rubrics containing at least two out of the four remedies Sec, Hura, Curare and Iod. The resultant list was then sorted, with the smallest rubrics coming first.

Mind; dreams; walking, of; ruins, among

Extremities; uncover, inclination to

Extremities; gangrene; leg

Mind; tears; himself

Mind; company; aversion to; avoids the sight of people

Vertigo; old people, in

Mind; tears; things

Mind; suicidal disposition; throwing himself from; height, a

Skin; warts; withered

Mind; travel; desire to

Mind; kill, desire to

Mind; contemptuous

Mind; destructiveness

Syphilitic Miasm:

Remedies selected for repertory search were: Merc, Aur, Lach, Syph and Hep Sulph. The list of rubrics was sorted with at least three of these remedies:

Mind; discontented, displeased, dissatisfied; always

Abdomen; abscess; inguinal region

Mind; moral affections; criminal, disposition to become a, without remorse

Mind; weary of life; perspiration, during

Mouth; ulcers; palate; syphilitic

Nose; sunken nose

Eye; injected; cornea

Face; ulcers; chin

Skin; abscess; hard to mature, give

Skin; ulcers; warmth; amel.

Skin; ulcers; heat; amel.

Skin; ulcers; painful; margins

Mouth; ulcers; base; lardaceous

Nose; inflammation; bones

Generalities; wounds; sudden disappearance of, by metastasis

Extremities; gangrene; threatened, with blue parts

Mind; impulse, morbid

Mind; anxiety; suicidal disposition, with

Skin; warts; syphilitic

Mind; suicidal disposition; perspiration, during.

F. SAMPLE CASE

By Melissa Burch, CCH

CASE of YOUNG WOMAN with SINUS PROBLEMS	*ANALYSIS*
Homeopath: Why don't we get started, okay?	
Client: Okay.	
So the main problem is...	
My sinus problems.	*Simple Chief Complaint – we see if it holds.*
Okay, so tell me everything you can about your sinus problems.	
I'm very stuffy, <u>constantly running</u>. Sometimes yellow-green. It's like sinus pressure, up here (*HG, hand gesture*). Sometimes it helps if I push on my eyebrows. I can feel it draining. My ears are always stuffed. It makes me tired. I sound weird (*her voice*) I don't know what else.	
Okay, I'll give you a little bit about how this works. I'm going to keep asking you the same questions, and you're going to tell me more and more. You're going to tell me more about your sinus problems than you've ever told anybody. So just describe it some more...it's constantly runny, it's stuffy, it's like this sinus pressure, it's better if you press on the eyebrows. What else?	*Explain Process.*
Sometimes my ears are full. Sometimes my jaw hurts. <u>My teeth feel like they're going to</u>	*Local Sensations.* *Delusion Language.*

CASE of YOUNG WOMAN with SINUS PROBLEMS	ANALYSIS
fall out or something (*HG – squeezing hand motion*). I have never really thought about my sinuses this much. I don't know. Just very stuffed—always stuffed. Like there is no relief from it. It keeps me up at night. I go through lots of tissues a day. I literally blow my nose like a hundred times. <u>It's non-stop.</u> It's in my throat (*HG*), like I always have something there. <u>It's a drip.</u> I have really itchy eyes (*same squeezing HG*). I have chronic sinusitis, so the doctor put me on prednazone and other medications. But nothing works. Do I have to think of more?	*HG repeats twice with Teeth and with Eyes – watch this.*
Well, you said it's like your teeth are going to fall out, it's like this drippy thing, it's something like this (HG). Just a little bit more about this (HG), the drippy quality, it feels like your teeth are going to fall out, it's running all the time. Just give me more.	*Picked up Repeated HG and Delusion Language and repeat this back to client to urge her forward.*
This is really hard. <u>I just want to keep saying constant.</u> Sore. Full. Pressure. Headaches. It makes me temperamental, I think. Just when I'm tired. It actually hurts now. Like here (*HG*), too, on my cheeks.	*How she Experiences her Chief Complaint of Sinus Issues is this that it is Constant, Non-Stop, Always, Chronic..............* *This Perception of her CC gives us clues to the Miasm.*
So describe this hurt now.	
It's a throbbing pain, again, <u>constant.</u> <u>Like someone is sitting on my face.</u> My nose <u>always</u> hurts, too, and it is very sensitive to touch. (*Same HG*)	*Delusion Language.*
So it's this like someone is sitting on your face, this sensitivity.	
Right. <u>Constant Pressure.</u> It is very sensitive.	

CASE of YOUNG WOMAN with SINUS PROBLEMS	ANALYSIS
It hurts. Like here, in the center of my forehead.	
You're doing good. So just describe what it's like for you to experience someone sitting on your face. Just how you experience this.	*Encourage and go to the Delusion to move her forwards. Trying to listen and find the Vital Expression.*
Crushing. Draining. Tiring. Again, the pressure. And just painful. It hurts.	*Local Sensation.*
It's constant, it's crushing, it's draining…	*Repeating back Local Sensation and Miasm words.*
Maybe like drilling (*same HG*), just always deeper and deeper. I'm trying to think of other things.	*Another Delusion.*
You're doing great. Just like drilling deeper and deeper. Just use more…more ways to describe the same thing.	*Still looking for the Vital Expression -- it appears to be the Repeated Hand Gesture….*
I'm just trying to think about it.	
Whatever comes to mind. You've described it really well. It's like pressure, it's draining, it's throbbing. It's like someone is sitting on your face, like your teeth are going to fall out…	*Repeating Back ALL the Language and Images and let HER Choose what to follow.*
Yes. It's just constant. It's almost like a bowling ball.	
So what's the bowling ball?	
It's just hard (*HG – open hands in front of her face*). Like pressure, like someone slamming into your face with a bowling ball. All the	*Again – another Delusion and more repetition of the Miasm Language of "all the time."*

CASE of YOUNG WOMAN with SINUS PROBLEMS	ANALYSIS
time.	
So again, very good. What's this, this constant, this feeling of someone sitting on your face, this bowling ball?	*Urging her to give the Experience of the Delusion.*
Yeah, just like "boom." Just knocking me out. Like really tired, napping all the time, constantly awake at night. Tossing, turning. Annoying . Pause...................... Aggressive (*HG*), pressure. My eyes will swell up so I can't see. I can't put my contacts in, so that sucks, because I really don't like wearing glasses. Lots of green goo from my eyes, lots of puss, tears often come out. I think I talk loud because I can't hear myself. Just like heavy, like hard, and it feels kind of hot. Just constant. I just keep wanting to say that word.	*Delusion with Energy.* *Emotion Language.* *Local Sensation.*
So it's constant, it's annoying. It can be hot. It's like pressure, it's like a big bowling ball slammed into your face, someone sitting on your face, just a bit more...	*Repeating Back her Language.* *The Homeopath is missing the importance of the one point the client repeats again and again -- this Constant.*
I hate how it affects my energy. It sucks. But, I mean, what can I do? Well, hopefully something. But it's just lousy. I hate it. I feel like I'm at a shrink or something because I'm going to start crying. I just feel like I'm an emotional wreck. I just hate it, I really do. It really affects my life and it sucks. And I feel so tired all the time and I hate that feeling, I really do. I'm sorry. I feel bad.	*Emotional Level.*
No, you're doing fine, you're doing beautifully. Because the way homeopathy works is, as you see, your emotions are connected to this feeling, the constancy, the pressure. All of these things are connected and there is another level to go	*Explaining the Process. The Homeopath has not been able to identify the Vital Expression.*

CASE of YOUNG WOMAN with SINUS PROBLEMS	ANALYSIS
to, to make a very deep prescription. And actually, you have given a lot of information, but there are different levels of prescriptions and we could pick one even now, because you have given a lot of information. But let's go to another level which connects the feeling of this constant tiredness, the sadness, and the pressure, as if someone was sitting on your face, like a bowling ball slamming. Just a bit more about what you experience with this tiredness, this constancy, that it sucks.	
I really don't know what else to say about it.	
How do you experience this constant tiredness?	
How do I experience it? <u>Daily</u>. <u>Every minute</u>. <u>It just never goes away—it's always there</u>. <u>I can't even remember a time when it wasn't there</u>. It makes me feel so bad. I have good energy, it's just that I get so tired. And I don't know what else I can do. How many more stupid things can I take for this? <u>And it just doesn't stop</u>. I mean, my nose is <u>always</u> stuffy, but it can get worse too. Like if I go into a horse barn or something. It just immediately...sometimes my lips swell.	*The case seems to just be about the Disease State and the Experience of it being Constant, Daily, Every Minute, Non Stop, Always.*
Immediately, what happens when it goes immediately?	
My eyes puff up and run, my lips can swell and get really itchy (*HG- same squeezing one as earlier*).	
What is this (HG)?	
This (HG)?	

CASE of YOUNG WOMAN with SINUS PROBLEMS	ANALYSIS
Well, you've used it a lot (HG). Like it's itchy, or it's drippy. What's this (HG) that you're trying to describe with your hands?	*Ask about the Hand Gesture and it doesn't really open the case so a good hint that it is not the Vital Expression.*
This pain.	
Okay, good.	
And pressure. It's just that I can't do certain things. I'm <u>limited</u>. And I hate being <u>limited</u>. Like I can't hang out with friends who have cats and I won't date a guy who has a cat because of my allergies because I'll swell up and not be able to see him and look gross.	*More Miasm Language.*
This pressure feeling, just more about the feeling of this pressure, like with the eyes. The pain is like a pressure. Just describe that a little bit more.	
I don't know. I just keep on saying <u>constant</u>. Like <u>constant pain and constantly there</u>. <u>It just never gives me a break</u>. And it doesn't help that I have a dog, but I won't give him up or anything. <u>It's just always there</u>. And it hurts. It's painful. It just sucks.	*The Client is telling the Homeopath that the Vital Expression is this CONSTANT.* *If we look back, the answer to every question and the consistent idea she repeats back to every inquiry is this "Constant."*
Ah.....so it's really the constant aspect that's bothering you.	
<u>Yes! It doesn't give me a break. It doesn't.</u>	
So it's as if what? What doesn't give you a break? Just whatever comes to mind.	
Just breathing. Like I can't breathe normally.	

CASE of YOUNG WOMAN with SINUS PROBLEMS	ANALYSIS
I just feel <u>limited</u> in everything because I can't breathe through my nose. It's a lousy feeling, it is. I snore because of it.	
So more about this feeling of being limited in everything, just what that is for you...	*Picking Up Miasm words and repeating back. Miasm is Obviously Sycotic and the Sensation of the Miasm seems to be the Overwhelming Sensation of the Case.*
Again, it's like a <u>limitation</u>, like I can't do certain things because I can't breathe right. And I am so stuffy, I am trying to gasp air into my mouth. It's just uncomfortable for me to be out and about with people, but I'm so social so it's hard for me not to go out. I just hate that <u>drippy</u>, like I <u>always</u> have to blow my nose every five minutes. I sniffle <u>constantly</u>.	
You're doing great. A little bit more of this feeling of limitation, of you can't do certain things, being social...	*The Case is all about Her Feeling due to the Disease and the Overwhelming Sensation is this Constancy.*
I wouldn't go to a club last weekend because I was like, "No, my nose is stuffy, it's going to run, I'm going to have to carry tissues." <u>I hate blowing my nose in public</u>. I blow my nose really loud. Because it's <u>always</u> full, I'm <u>constantly</u> trying to clear it out (*HG – sweeping downwards*).	
What is this (HG)? Just this (HG).	
<u>Just like the mucus, and junk</u>, and just getting it out of my body. I'm so sick of it. And I don't know where all of it comes from. I try to drink plenty of water, but it just creates this mass amount of mucus. So I let it limit my social life and my life. And I just hate that.	

CASE of YOUNG WOMAN with SINUS PROBLEMS	ANALYSIS
And I feel like I can't control it.	
So, a bit more about this feeling that it limits your social life.	
Well, I'm still really social, but like my friend Steve, who I love, constantly makes fun of me. He's like, "you sound like…" and then he pinches his nose and makes fun of me. It's just <u>always</u> there. <u>People notice it</u> and it makes me uncomfortable to talk about it, but it's something that <u>I talk about every single day</u>. Because I don't have a choice. <u>Because people know.</u> So I just wish that people didn't have to hear me sound stuffy <u>all the time</u>. I would just like one day where I could breathe and not feel <u>mucusy</u> and <u>gross</u>. I just want to be able to breathe through my nose. It's <u>constantly</u> red and irritated and dry. I just hate it.	*All the Case is the Constancy of the Disease State and how it Limits her Life. All the Case is the Experience of the Disease State and the Question of Why am I in this State and Different from Everyone Else.* *It is Only about Disease and Health and the Predominant Experience is of the Miasm.* **THIS IS A NOSODE CASE and the NOSODE is MEDORRHINUM – the NOSODE of the SYCOTIC MIASM.**
You're doing great. Just a little bit more about this constant feeling, that you can't breathe, it's mucusy, it's gross, it's limiting, it's constant.	*Repeating Back the Vital Expression of Constant with her descriptions.*
<u>It smells bad.</u> <u>If it gets infected, I can smell it.</u> <u>It's just nasty.</u> And I know at that time, obviously, I need medicine. I just feel like the doctors don't take it seriously. I've tried the allergy shots and they didn't work. <u>I've tried so many things and I'm just sick of nothing working.</u> I really am. I am so sick of it.	*This is actually Source Language creeping in…….* *Nosode Kingdom Sensation:* *Try Everything to Correct the Problem and Regain Health.*
I just want you to describe now, one more time from the beginning what happens to you. You've explained it very well, I just want you to sort-of put it all together for me.	*Checking the Premise that this is actually a Nosode Case by having her go back to the beginning and put the pieces together and listening for anything that doesn't fit.*

CASE of YOUNG WOMAN with SINUS PROBLEMS	ANALYSIS
Like what?	
What happens to you, how do you experience this constancy, the dripping, the pressure, the limitations? Or give a really good example of when it was the most intense for you when it happened.	
There are so many to choose from. But like the other night, I don't know what I did, but I literally just rubbed my eye and before I knew it my eyes were out to here—they were <u>sealed</u> shut. I don't even know what I touched, maybe there was dust, I don't know. But literally, my nose was like an <u>instant faucet</u> *(HG of sweeping down)*, it just kept going, my eyes <u>swelled</u> shut, and my nose was just really <u>runny</u> and <u>gross</u> and I didn't do anything. I probably walked by something and it had perfume on it. So just little things like that trigger it. I could be anywhere. It's just <u>embarrassing</u>. I hate it, I really do.	*Listening for Nosode Kingdom Language and even hints of Source Languge........*
Just a little bit about last night when your eyes just sealed shut. A little bit more about how you experienced that.	
Well, I could feel it coming, so I tried not to touch my eyes. I put eye-drops in. I put cloths on. But they got all <u>mucusy and yellow</u>, and I really couldn't see at all, so I had to lie down. And I was like, "I don't have time for this." I just…I don't have time. And I can't go out because I can't see, I can't drive, and I'm just <u>stuck</u> there thinking, "hopefully tomorrow morning when I wake up I will be able to see and my eyes will be less swollen." Like I'll go to work and I'll wear my glasses if I've had a bad night and my eyes are <u>swollen</u> and sore and red. And makeup only <u>hides</u> so much. It just sucks that I can't see. I can't	*Sycotic Miasm words keep coming up – Stuck, Hides, Embarrassing, Daily/Constant.*

CASE of YOUNG WOMAN with SINUS PROBLEMS	*ANALYSIS*
breathe. It's such a pain. I don't know why it has to be on a <u>daily basis</u>. <u>It's every single day</u>.	
You're doing good. What is it like for you not to be able to see?	
It's horrible. I mean, my brothers laugh at me, and I feel trapped. I'm <u>stuck</u>. I can't go out, I can't drive my car. I can't do anything. I'll go outside, but to do what, just sit there and hope the fresh air helps? But then, air has allergens too. Everything just makes it worse, and <u>there's nothing I can do that makes it better</u>. I literally just go to bed and hope that in the morning it's better. And sometimes it is and the swelling goes down, but it's like it will happen again for something else. One day it's perfume, one day it's the dog, if he picked up grass or something. I just never know what is going to trigger it—or when. I don't know. I do hate it, though.	*Sycotic Miasm – Stuck and Nothing I can do.....*
And this feeling of being trapped and you can't see, what's that like for you?	
Boring and lonely and I'm just there. I can't watch TV, I can't instant message on the computer, I don't want to talk on the phone because my eyes are swollen and my nose is <u>like a fountain</u>. I can't communicate. I yell at my parents for no reason. I just get miserable when I'm like that and I take it out on everybody around me. Like I blame them. I know it's not their fault, of course not. And then I feel bad later for that. But they don't understand what it's like and they <u>constantly</u> tell me, "just go get your nose fixed." And I tried it, it didn't work. <u>I can't help it</u>. I don't know why it does it. But, you know, <u>they have no idea how lucky they are that they don't have to deal with this</u>. And they just don't get	*The Whole Experience is Just the Drama of the Constancy of the Disease State.* *Emotional Level Coming in.* *Nosode Kingdom Language:* *"Me" different from everyone else.*

CASE of YOUNG WOMAN with SINUS PROBLEMS	ANALYSIS
it. They really don't.	
So what would it be like then to be lucky enough...?	
<u>Just being able to do everything that normal people</u> do everyday and not have to think about carrying tissues or allergy spray or eye drops or any of that stuff. You know, they might have other health issues, but at least they can breathe and see and not sniffle <u>every two seconds</u>. And I don't know, I just feel sorry for myself. And it's stupid, but...I don't know. <u>Everyone has their flaw</u>, I guess.	*Nosode Kingdom Sensation and Language:* *I'm not Normal – I am Diseased --I'm Flawed.*
Okay, good. A little bit more about this not being able to breathe and see. You're doing great, because everything is putting it together. Just a little bit more. What's it like not to be able to breathe or see?	
I don't know. I have asthma too. So, when I was a kid, I couldn't breathe because I had asthma attacks and stuff. Now I'm better, but it just, I don't know, I freak out. I get scared. I don't know, I just figure <u>something is wrong with me</u>, you know, <u>what is creating all of this mucus and gross stuff that keeps coming</u>? And where the hell does it come from? I don't know.	*Nosode Kingdom Sensation:* *Something Wrong within Me.*
So that's the feeling, all this stuff is coming?	
Yeah, <u>it just keeps coming. It never stops. It really doesn't</u>. Like I can't breathe through my nose ever. Like I can't even tell you the last time I was able to sniffle and not feel <u>mucussy</u>, <u>wet</u>, <u>gross</u> stuff up there. I mean, I don't even remember. I really don't. It's been a long,	

CASE of YOUNG WOMAN with SINUS PROBLEMS	ANALYSIS
long time.	
Okay, you're doing something really different here, okay? This feeling that it never stops, this mucussy, it keeps coming, this gross, just, in the imagination, what is this? You've described it very well. But just now, whatever comes to mind from this, something that keeps coming, it's mucussy, it's gross, it's constant…	*Now Go to Source off the Vital Expression of Constant.*
You know, like putty stuff that looks like boogers? That's the form. *(squeezing HG from the beginning of the case)* I just feel like it's all up there *(sweeping down HG)*. It's like this plasticky, I don't know. Is that what you're looking for?	*Listening for Source Language: Putty, Boogers, Plasticky.* *Same HG appear from earlier in the case which is a nice confirmation.*
Yeah, perfect. Exactly.	*Encourage her.*
Just like that.	
You're doing this (HG). What is this (HG)?	
It's <u>gooey</u> (HG), <u>drippy (HG)</u>, everywhere. It starts like that and <u>just shoots everywhere</u>.	*Source Language: Gooey, Drippy, Shoots Everywhere.*
Okay, great, what's this gooey, that shoots like everywhere. Just whatever comes to mind.	
It's that <u>big booger</u>. <u>Like rubber cement</u>. Just a <u>waterfall</u>. <u>Like an explosion</u>. Umm, I don't know, <u>like a river or something</u>. <u>Like it starts one place and goes</u>.	*Lots of Delusion coming up at this Sensation/Source Level. This "Starts one place and goes" is the Experience of the Previous Delusions.*

CASE of YOUNG WOMAN with SINUS PROBLEMS	ANALYSIS
Great. Just focus on this a little bit. Something that's like this booger. It's plasticky, it's gooey, it's like rubber cement, it shoots, it's a waterfall, it's an explosion. Just whatever comes. Like a river that comes and goes. Whatever comes to mind. It doesn't have to be about your sinus problems. Just whatever comes to mind with this.	*Repeat Back EVERYTHING.*
Umm. <u>I want to say like epidemic.</u> Something like a word like that, <u>something that just keeps spreading</u>. I don't know. I'm really stuffy now. But I won't blow my nose, because <u>I won't do that in public, which is another weird thing</u>.	*Sensation Language of the Nosode Kingdom: Epidemic, Spreading.* *Sycotic Miasm: Won't do in Public.*
So, more about this booger, this plasticky, it shoots, it's like an explosion, like rubber cement, a waterfall, a river that starts one place and goes, like an epidemic that keeps spreading.	
I don't know what else. I don't know. More <u>like a stream than a river</u>, (HG) I guess, the kind that has little streams off it, because <u>it goes not just to one place</u>. Umm. I don't know, <u>I just keep picturing the green booger and it's really grossing me out</u>.	
Okay, just describe everything you can about that green booger. Whatever you can.	
It's <u>mushy, slimy, unappealing, gooey</u>. I don't know, what's the texture? <u>Mushy</u>, I guess. Umm, <u>big</u>. It's like <u>bumps</u>. I don't know, I just feel like it has <u>bumps</u>. I don't know. It's just <u>constant</u>. It <u>stretches</u>. I don't know what else it does. It <u>sticks</u>. What else does it do? I don't know. I don't know. I have a headache.	*Source Language. The "Constant" comes back so it confirms we are in the right place.* *Beautiful description of the Source Material used to prepare Medorrhinum.*

CASE of YOUNG WOMAN with SINUS PROBLEMS	ANALYSIS
I think you did a good job.	Remedy: medorrhinum
	Potency: 30C

Overview: Client describes fact level with sinuses in great detail. Homeopath feeds her back delusion language to take her deeper. Client answers every question with sycotic miasm language of "constant" which is also the VE. Case is all about her feelings due to the disease and the overwhelming sensation of constancy and how it limits her life.

Chief Complaint: Sinus trouble

Vital Expression: Constant

Some questions the homeopath asks:
Well, you said it's like your teeth are going to fall out, it's like this drippy thing, it's something like this (HG). Just a little bit more about this (HG), the drippy quality, it feels like your teeth are going to fall out, it's running all the time. Just give me more.
You're doing good. So just describe what it's like for you to experience someone sitting on your face. Just how you experience this.
Whatever comes to mind. You've described it really well. It's like pressure, it's draining, it's throbbing. It's like someone is sitting on your face, like your teeth are going to fall out... Ah.....so it's really the constant aspect that's bothering you.
Okay, you're doing something really different here, okay? This feeling that it never stops, this mucousy, it keeps coming, this gross, just, in the imagination, what is this? You've described it very well. But just now, whatever comes to mind from this.
Great. Just focus on this a little bit. Something that's like this booger. It's plasticky, it's gooey, it's like rubber cement, it shoots, it's a waterfall, it's an explosion. Just whatever comes. Like a river that comes and goes. Whatever comes to mind. It doesn't have to be about your sinus problems. Just whatever comes to mind with this.

Kingdom Language:
Just constant. I just keep wanting to say that word.
How do I experience it? Daily. Every minute. It just never goes away—it's always there. I can't even remember a time when it wasn't there. It makes me feel so bad.
I just keep on saying constant. Like constant pain and constantly there. It just never gives me a break.
I've tried so many things and I'm just sick of nothing working.
I just figure something is wrong with me, you know, what is creating all of this mucus and gross stuff that keeps coming?
I want to say like epidemic. Something like a word like that, something that just keeps spreading.

Source Language:

Mucousy, yellow, runny, gunk. It smells bad. If it gets infected, I can smell it. It's just nasty. Mucousy, wet, gross stuff. Like putty stuff that looks like boogers. Plasticky. Gooey drippy, shoots everywhere.

It's mushy, slimy, unappealing, gooey. I don't know, what's the texture? Mushy, I guess. Umm, big. It's like bumps. I don't know, I just feel like it has bumps. I don't know. It's just constant. It stretches. I don't know what else it does. It sticks.

Energy Language:

HG squeezing

Miasm: Sycotic (the sensation of the miasm is the overwhelming sensation of the case)

Constant, non-stop, always, chronic... I just want to keep saying constant... All the time... I just feel limited in everything because I can't breathe through my nose...

I am limited. And I hate being limited... I hate blowing my nose in public... People notice it and it makes me uncomfortable to talk about it, but it's something that I talk about every single day. Because I don't have a choice. Because people know.

And makeup only hides so much... I don't know why it has to be on a daily basis. It's every single day... I mean, my brothers laugh at me, and I feel trapped. I'm stuck... Just being able to do everything that normal people do everyday... But I won't blow my nose, because I won't do that in public.

Remedy: Medorrhinum (nosode of the sycotic miasm)   **Dose:** 30c

G. HOMEWORK

Please submit three paper cases. Circle or highlight all the miasm language and identify, which miasm you think it is, as well as the level you think the patient is expressing the ideas.

For feedback you can send or email your homework to:

Melissa Burch, CCH
Inner Health, Inc.
175 Harvey Street, Unit 13
Cambridge, MA 02140 USA

617-491-3374

melissa@innerhealth.us

www.innerhealth.us

About Melissa Burch, CCH

Melissa Burch, CCH, co-founded The Catalyst School of Homeopathy with Christopher Beaver, CCH. She established live phone case supervision and clinics based on the Sensation Method.

She created a unique homeopathic phone referral service with a homeopath team approach. She is president of Inner Health, Inc., which produces numerous online and onsite courses for homeopaths, homeopathic patients and people interested in alternative medicine. She produced the first Radio Series on Homeopathy.

She was the Master Homeopath for the proving of Stoichactis Kenti Sea Anemone. She co-wrote and published the five part "Vital Sensation Manual." Ms. Burch worked with Dr. Nandita Shah at Quiet Healing Center in South India for over a year and half. She graduated from the School of Homeopathy New York, directed by Jo Daly, and the New York School of Homeopathy, directed by Robert Stewart.

About Inner Health, Inc.

Inner Health (IH) provides homeopathic services to the general public and to the homeopathic community. IH is a leader in establishing the highest quality of services in the complementary and alternative medical field through its education, practitioners, workshops and services.

IH's vision is to make homeopathy a household word. Our goal is to identify IH in the consumer's mind as the place to go for the best, natural deep healing on all level—mental, emotional, physical and spiritual; and to create a demand for homeopathy and in particular for Certified IH Homeopaths, through our innovative, educational and creative marketing materials.

Training

IH provides basic and post-graduate training for homeopaths to develop reliable and better results in their practices by following the IH Approach—a systematic way of case taking and analysis based on the Sensation Method—and by implementing the IH System, which includes case management protocols, scripts and information, client business services and marketing.

Homeopaths have the opportunity to train and become Certified IH Homeopaths through workshops, supervision and educational materials. Combined with our own extensive marketing of IH and the IH approach to homeopathy, which results in constant referrals to Certified IH Homeopaths, IH Homeopaths will have a unique and wonderful opportunity to develop themselves as professional homeopaths, heal others, share clinical information with the homeopathic community, be well paid and have excellent systems to guide them to provide the highest care to the client.

Printed in Great Britain
by Amazon.co.uk, Ltd.,
Marston Gate.